CONQUER YOUR
NEGATIVE THOUGHTS

CONQUER YOUR NEGATIVE THOUGHTS

THE SECRET TO EMOTIONAL FREEDOM AND HAPPINESS

DANIEL G. AMEN, MD

#1 NEW YORK TIMES BESTSELLING AUTHOR

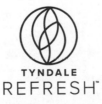

TYNDALE
REFRESH™

Think Well. Live Well. Be Well.

Visit Tyndale online at tyndale.com.

Visit Daniel G. Amen, MD, at danielamenmd.com.

Published in association with the literary agency of WordServe Literary Group, www.wordserveliterary.com.

For information about special discounts for bulk purchases, please contact Tyndale House Publishers at csresponse@tyndale.com, or call 1-855-277-9400.

ISBN 978-1-4964-5764-6

Printed in the United States of America

29   28   27   26   25   24   23
7   6   5   4   3

Contents

Introduction *1*

Chapter 1 Understanding Your Negative Thoughts *5*

Chapter 2 You Are What You Think *33*

Chapter 3 The Power of Positivity *81*

Appendix A How Challenging 100 of Your Worst
Thoughts Can Change Your Life *121*

Appendix B Bible Verses to Help Conquer Negative
Thoughts *137*

About the Author *145*

Notes *151*

Introduction

A thought is harmless unless we believe it.
It's not our thoughts, but the attachment to our thoughts,
that causes suffering. Attaching to a thought means
believing that it's true, without inquiring. A belief is a
thought that we've been attaching to, often for years.

BYRON KATIE, *Loving What Is:*
Four Questions That Can Change Your Life

ACCORDING TO A 2015 STUDY from Microsoft, the human attention span is eight seconds.[1] A goldfish's attention span has been estimated at nine seconds. Human development seems to be going the wrong way. With modern technology stealing our attention spans and directing our minds to the will of corporate America, disciplining the habits of our moment-by-moment thoughts is an essential skill for achieving happiness and purpose. Our gadget addiction is feeding an old tendency of the human brain to be scattered, unfocused, and controlled by negativity and fear.

Plus, it is making us feel worse.[2] People who have the most screen time (TV, texting, video games) have a higher incidence of feeling unhappy.

These habits can lead to *monkey mind*, a term that describes a mind that is unsettled, restless, indecisive, and uncontrollable. Monkey mind was described by Siddhartha Gautama (Buddha) in the sixth century BC, but it applies today more than ever. He said, "Just as a monkey swinging through the trees grabs one branch and lets it go only to seize another, so, too, that which is called thought, mind, or consciousness arises and disappears continually both day and night."

Thoughts that *you allow* to circle again and again in your mind build ruts or roads in the brain, making the thoughts more likely to dominate and control your life.

Fortunately, you aren't doomed to feel down when life doesn't go your way. You can learn how to consistently generate positive feelings no matter your age, income, or situation.

As a psychiatrist, I've written about anxiety, depression, bipolar disorder, attention deficit hyperactivity disorder (ADHD), aging, violence, obesity, memory loss, love, parenting, and other important topics. Yet underlying the reasons most people come to see us at Amen Clinics is the fact that they are unhappy. Helping people be happier day to day is at the core of getting and staying mentally and physically healthy.

Extensive research has shown that happiness is associated with a lower heart rate, lower blood pressure, and overall heart health. Happier people get fewer infections, have lower cortisol levels (the hormone of stress), and fewer aches and pains. Happy people tend to live longer, have better relationships, and be more successful in their careers. Plus happiness is contagious because happier people tend to make others happier.

One of my favorite short videos that I encourage all of my patients to watch is by author and talk show host Dennis Prager. In "Why Be Happy?" he suggests that happiness is a moral obligation. He says:

> Whether or not you're happy, and most
> importantly, whether or not you act
> happy is about altruism, not selfishness—
> because it is about how we affect others'

lives. . . . Ask anybody who was raised by an unhappy parent whether or not happiness is a moral issue, and I assure you the answer will be "yes." It is no fun being raised by an unhappy parent, or being married to an unhappy person, or being the parent of an unhappy child, or working with an unhappy coworker.[3]

Over the course of the next few chapters, I am going to show you how to identify, understand, and conquer the negative thoughts that are stealing your happiness and teach you how to retrain your brain to focus on the positive and improve your overall quality of life.

Ready? Good. Let's get started.

CHAPTER 1

UNDERSTANDING YOUR NEGATIVE THOUGHTS

Dark thoughts in the mind are not "you," but are false messages from the brain. And because you are not your brain, you don't have to listen to them.

JEFFREY M. SCHWARTZ, MD,
author of *You Are Not Your Brain*

IT HAD BEEN A REALLY TOUGH DAY at the office. I had seen four suicidal patients, two teens who had run away from home, and two couples who hated each other. As if this wasn't bad enough, that evening, when I arrived home and walked into the kitchen, I was greeted by an ant infestation. The little critters were everywhere, coming out of light sockets and spaces between the flooring and the walls. I even found ants in the pantry crawling into cereal boxes. Construction in our neighborhood had disturbed the earth, and the ants were looking for a new residence.

Apparently, word had gotten out to a sizable ant colony that the pickings were good in the Amen home.

As I wet paper towels and began wiping up the horde of ants, the acronym ANT came to me—Automatic Negative Thought. Acronyms had been part of my life since medical school, helping me remember the 50,000 new terms I was learning. As I thought about my patients that day, I realized that, just like my kitchen, they were also infested with ANTs that were robbing them of their joy and stealing their happiness. A bizarre image came to me of ANTs crawling on top of their heads and out of their eyes, noses, and ears. The ANTs were setting up residence inside my patients' minds. The next day I brought a can of ant spray to work and placed it on my coffee table. As I started to talk about the concept with my patients, they understood it right away.

ANTs are thoughts that pop into your mind uninvited. They make you feel mad, sad, worried, or upset. And most of the time they're not even true!

Think of automatic

negative thoughts as you would the ants that might bother a couple at a romantic picnic. One negative thought, like one ant at a picnic, is not a big problem. Two or three automatic negative thoughts, like two or three ants at a picnic, become a bit more irritating. Twenty or 30 automatic negative thoughts, like 20 or 30 ants at a picnic, may cause the couple to pick up and leave. The more you allow the ANTs to stick around in your head, the more they will "mate" with other ANTs and produce offspring that drive school failure, anxiety, depression, anger, work strife, relationship turmoil, and even obesity.

The nine different ANT species

About 10 years ago, the parents of 14-year-old Marcus brought him to see me because he was struggling with schoolwork and with his temper. At his previous school, Marcus "barely had to try" to get good grades; but after moving to a new school for the athletics, he found the more academically rigorous program challenging, and his grades declined. He had trouble focusing, was easily distracted, procrastinated, and took longer to complete assignments than ever before. A prior psychiatrist diagnosed him with attention deficit hyperactivity disorder (ADHD), but the stimulant medications Ritalin and Adderall made him angry and more depressed, and for the first time he started to complain of suicidal thoughts.

When I met Marcus, it was clear he struggled with many negative thoughts. He repeatedly referred to himself as stupid, and during our first session he told me,

"I hate school."
"I can never be as good as other kids."
"I'm a terrible person."
"I should try harder."
"I am not as smart as the other kids."
"I'll never go to college."
"I am a failure."
"My teachers hate me."
"It's my parents' fault for not letting me quit."

Over the years, therapists have identified nine different types of negative thought patterns that keep your mind off balance. I think of these as "species" of ANTs. They go by various names, but these are the ones I like to use:

1. All-or-Nothing ANTs

2. Just-the-Bad ANTs

3. Guilt-Beating ANTs

4. Labeling ANTs

5. Fortune-Telling ANTs

6. Mind-Reading ANTs

7. Blaming ANTs

8. Less-Than ANTs

9. If-Only and I'll-Be-Happy-When ANTs

In the course of our conversation, Marcus exhibited all of them. Let's take a closer look at each one.

All-or-Nothing ANTs. When Marcus told me, "I can never be as good as other kids," that was an example of an All-or-Nothing ANT. These sneaky ANTs attack whenever you think things are all good or all bad. They don't use words like *sometimes* or *maybe*. These ANTs think in absolute words that make situations *all good* or *all bad*. This is also called black-or-white thinking because it splits reality into light and dark, or good and bad, without acknowledging life's complexities, ambiguities, and nuances.

You know these ANTs are around whenever you think in words like *all, always, any, never, no one, nothing, everyone, every time*. These ANTs attack when you believe things are completely right or totally wrong, that people are either friends or enemies, that a day is perfect or terrible, or that you are a total success or a complete failure. These ANTs tell you that it is now or never, that everything that is not good is bad, that you are beautiful or ugly, that you love or hate someone, and so on.

I once saw the runner-up to the television show *The Biggest Loser*. He had lost over 100 pounds. Yet he was depressed because he saw himself as a complete failure since he did not finish first. He beat out many other contestants and literally lost the weight equivalent to a small adult.

All-or-Nothing ANTs make clear, rigid, and lasting distinctions often based on half-truths or lies. They reduce complex concepts into two opposing categories: good or bad. On the surface, these ANTs make you feel better about yourself because you can put people and actions into simple categories. Just open any political news feed and you'll see pundits putting the other side into the all-bad category.

It's easy to spot all-or-nothing thinkers as they tend to see only one side of a situation, ignore evidence to the contrary, and get into heated arguments with people who do not share their views. Yet this stinking thinking pattern obscures judgment, leads to bad decisions, decreases one's ability to understand the world, ruins relationships, and reduces the number of ways to solve problems.

Here's an example: At Amen Clinics we did the first and largest study on active and retired NFL players. More than half of our retired players were obese, which is very bad for the brain, so we ran a weight-loss group for athletes. One obese player told me that he was fat because he just didn't like any of the foods that were healthy for him. "Is that really true?" I asked. "You don't like any of them?" I then showed him a list of

50 brain healthy foods, and in fact, he liked about 60 percent of them. The All-or-Nothing ANTs were controlling his food choices and making him fat. Another example: I heard many All-or-Nothing ANTs from my patients as well as from people on social media while the country was in lockdown during the COVID-19 pandemic.

Here are examples of All-or-Nothing ANTs, including some of the more common pandemic-induced ANTs I heard:

"All of my freedom is being taken away from me during the pandemic."

"We're all going to get COVID-19."

"I am not a good father."

"No one cares about me."

"Nothing ever works out for me."

"I am an abject failure."

"I am not a good Christian."

"My boss is taking advantage of me."

"My husband is the devil incarnate."

"We had an argument. I think our relationship is over."

"I couldn't run a mile. I'll never be an athlete and should just quit working out."

"I don't want to talk to anyone anymore."

"My wife never listens to me."

"I thought I did a good report, but my boss asked me to make a few changes. I can't do anything right."

"I'm so bored; there's nothing to do."

Just-the-Bad ANTs. "I always hate school" is an example of one of Marcus's Just-the-Bad ANTs. Thousands of years ago, human minds were trained to focus on the negative because it kept people safe. Today, even though lions, tigers, and bears are not likely to eat you, your brain is still primed to pay attention to potential danger before focusing on anything positive.

To take advantage of our negative tendency, internet marketers feed us a nonstop stream of negative news to increase clicks and traffic to their sites. Have you noticed breaking news is pervasive and never good? Our society is infesting us with Just-the-Bad ANTs. These pesky creatures see only the bad in a situation and ignore anything good! Unless you manage your internet usage, you are swamped with distressing news about terror attacks, political scandals, fires, floods, hurricanes, global warming, mass shootings, murder-suicides, executions, and more. Negative news sells, and since we are always being sold something for the financial gain of others, we are flooded with toxic thoughts.

Just-the-Bad ANTs also zoom their beady eyes in on your mistakes and problems. They fill your head with failure, frustration, sadness, and fear. These ANTs can take virtually any positive experience and taint it with negativity. They are the judge, jury, and executioner of any new experiences, new relationships, and new habits.

Focusing on the negative releases brain chemicals that make you feel bad and that reduce brain activity in the prefrontal cortex, the area involved with self-control, judgment, and planning. This increases the odds of your making bad choices, such as ordering a third drink, eating a bowlful of chips, or staying up so late updating your social networking site that you wake up exhausted and need to guzzle caffeine to get going.

Some examples of Just-the-Bad ANTs include thoughts like these:

The world is more dangerous than ever.

*I went to the gym and did a hard workout,
but the guy on the bike next to me was
talking the whole time, so I'm never going
back there.*

*I gave a presentation at work, and even though
many people told me they loved it, one
person fell asleep during my talk, so it must
have really been terrible.*

*I only got into the college of my second choice.
I failed.*

The economy is never going to get better.

I love people who don't love me back.

*I got together with an old friend, but she
showed up 10 minutes late for lunch,
so I'm not going to call her again.*

*I cut back my caffeine intake from ten cups
of coffee a day to two, but I wanted to get
down to no coffee by now, so I should just
quit trying.*

*I got into our vacation home an hour late and
the lights were out. What a disaster!*

*My record debuted at #2 on the Billboard
charts; I am so disappointed.*

*Our city league baseball team finished second;
the whole season was a waste of time.*

*My son got four As on his report card but also
two Bs. I'm so disappointed.*

*I've been good with my diet all week, but
because I cheated on Friday, it ruined
everything.*

Guilt-Beating ANTs. With Guilt-Beating ANTs, motivation comes from moral beatings you received from others, such as parents and authority figures: "You should have done that. You ought to do this. You mustn't think like that ever again." Whenever you think in words like *should, must, ought,* or *have to,* your brain is beating you up with guilt.

Growing up Roman Catholic and going to parochial schools through ninth grade, I had to pass Guilt 101 and Advanced Guilt. Only kidding—but *should* and *shouldn't* were common words when I was growing up. Of course, there are many important *should* and *shouldn't* thoughts, but in my 30-plus years as a psychiatrist, I've found that guilt is generally not a helpful motivator of behavior. It often backfires and can be counterproductive to your goals.

When Marcus told me he "should try harder in school," that statement didn't help him actually do better. In fact, to Marcus, it seemed the harder he tried, the worse he performed.

Here are some examples of Guilt-Beating ANTs:

> *I'm not a good son because I do not call my dad. I should do better.*
> *I should Zoom or FaceTime with my parents more often.*
> *I have to give up sugar.*
> *I must start counting my calories.*
> *I ought to exercise more.*
> *I should be more giving.*
> *I'm ashamed of the sexual experiences I had as a preteen. I should not have done those things.*
> *My struggles are my fault. I should be better.*
> (This is also a Blaming ANT.)
> *I'm selfish for seeking help. I shouldn't have to do it.* (This is also a Labeling ANT.)

*I should quit because all the work problems are
    my fault.* (This is also a Blaming ANT.)
I feel guilty for taking time for myself.
*I should be able to beat this depression without
    medicine.*
I should not have made this move to a new job.
I must do better in school.
I should be a better wife/husband.

Labeling ANTs. Whenever you label yourself or
someone else with a negative term, you inhibit
your ability to take an honest look at the situation. When Marcus thought, *I am an idiot*, he
lumped himself in with all of the people he ever
thought were idiots, which damaged his self-
esteem and his ability to make progress in his
life. Labeling ANTs strengthen negative pathways in the brain, making the ruts deeper and
their walls thicker. These habitual ruts lead to
troubled behaviors. If, for example, you label
yourself as "lazy," then why bother trying to do
better in school or at work? The Labeling ANT
will cause you to give up before you try, and it
will keep you stuck in your old ways. Examples
of Labeling ANTs include:

He's a jerk
I'm lazy.
I'm a loser.
She's cold.
I'm a lousy businessperson.
I sound like an idiot.
I'm fat.
I'm evil because I hurt a cat when I was eight.
I'm selfish.
She's weak.
You're weird.
You're too gullible.
You're a bad son.
He's a narcissist.

The problem with Labeling ANTs is that they trick you into thinking that it is impossible to change. You are what you are.

Even positive labels can be harmful. I tell parents, for example, never to praise children for being smart; praise them instead for working hard. When you tell children they are smart, they become more performance oriented and assume that intelligence cannot be improved. If they start to struggle with a new task, they may feel "not smart" and give up. But if you praise children for working hard, when they come up against a difficult task, they will persist because "they work hard."

Fortune-Telling ANTs. Don't listen to these lying ANTs! Fortune-Telling ANTs think they can see what is going to happen in the future, but all they really do is think up bad stuff that makes you upset. They creep into your mind and predict the future with fear. Of course, it is helpful to prepare for potential problems, but if you spend all your time focused on a fearful future, you will be filled with anxiety. Marcus's anxiety was driven by his Fortune-Telling ANTs, such as *I will fail school . . . I'll never go to college . . . I will be a failure.*

Other examples of the thoughts from this deceiver include:

> *Nothing will ever be "normal" again after the pandemic. Everything will be worse.*
> *I'm doomed to be unemployed for years.*
> *Inflation is never going to come down.*
> *I'm going to get sick and die.*

I'll become homeless.
My children will also have a mental illness.
I'll die without him.
If I give that presentation, I'll have a panic attack.
None of my investments will pay off.
I'll look stupid when I talk.
I won't be able to buy a house.
I'll never exercise again.
I'll never be good at public speaking.
My friend killed himself; I am doomed.
My kids will get a better dad if I die.

Predicting the worst in a situation causes an immediate rise in heart and breathing rates and can make you feel anxious. It can trigger cravings for sugar or refined carbs and make you feel as if you need to eat to calm your anxiety. What makes Fortune-Telling ANTs even worse is that your mind is so powerful, it can make what you imagine happen. When you think you will sprain your ankle, for example, that thought may deactivate the cerebellum, making you more clumsy and likely to get hurt. Similarly, if you are convinced you won't get a good night's sleep or find a new relationship, you will be less likely to engage in the behaviors that might make it so.

Mind-Reading ANTs. These ANTs are convinced they can see inside someone else's mind and know how others think and feel without even being told. They say things like "Everyone thinks I am stupid," or "They are laughing at me." When you're sure you know what others are thinking even though they have not told you and you have not asked them, you are feeding your Mind-Reading ANTs. When Marcus told me, "My teachers hate me," he was allowing this ANT to torture him. I have 25 years of education, and I can't tell what anyone else is thinking unless they tell me. A glance in your direction doesn't mean somebody is talking about you or mad at you. I tell people that a negative look from someone else may mean nothing more than that he or she is constipated! You just don't know.

I teach all my patients the "18-40-60 Rule," which says that when you are 18 you worry about what everyone thinks of you; when you are 40 you don't care what anyone thinks about you;

and when you are 60 you realize no one has been thinking about you at all. People spend their days worrying and thinking about themselves, not about you. Stop trying to read their minds. Examples include:

> *My dad thinks I'm weak.*
> *My boss doesn't like me.*
> *People think I'm fearful for wearing a mask in public.*
> *My friends think I won't be able to keep up with them on our hike.*
> *My father thinks I'll never amount to much.*
> *People think I'm dumb.*
> *People think I'm being treated for depression to get attention.*
> *People at work don't care about me.*
> *I can die, and people won't care.*
> *Everyone is disappointed in me.*
> *My mom doesn't think I measure up compared to my siblings.*
> *I frustrate all the people who know me.*
> *My wife would rather be with someone else.*
> *My pastor doesn't care about me.*
> *He thinks everyone else is an idiot.*

Blaming ANTs. When Marcus said, "It's my parents' fault for not letting me quit," he was allowing Blaming ANTs to take hold in his brain. Blaming ANTs always sing the same old sad song: *He did it! She did it! It's not my fault! It's your fault!* These ANTs don't want you to admit your mistakes or learn how to fix things and make them right; they want you to be a victim. Of all the ANTs, Blaming ANTs are the most toxic. I call them red ANTs, because they not only steal your happiness, but also drain you of your personal power. When you blame something or someone else for the problems in your life, you become a victim of circumstances who can't do anything to change the situation. Blame also starts a dangerous downhill slide that goes something like this:

Blames others
"It's your fault."
↓
Sees life as beyond personal control
"My life would be better if it weren't for . . ."
↓
Feels like a victim of circumstances
"If only that hadn't happened, then . . ."

↓

Gives up trying
"Nothing will ever go right for me. Why try?"

Blaming others temporarily rids yourself of feelings of guilt or responsibility. However, it also reinforces the idea that life is out of your control and that others can determine how life goes for you.

Psychiatrists have known for some time that the patients who do the worst in psychotherapy are the ones who take no personal responsibility for getting better. In fact, as early as Freud (1927), a major goal of psychotherapy has been increasing patients' sense of personal responsibility. Dr. Carl Rogers went so far as to develop a "personal responsibility" scale to predict those who would get better with treatment and those who would not.

Be honest and ask yourself if you have a tendency to say things like:

"It's their fault that the coronavirus kept spreading."
"It's your fault I failed because you didn't do enough to help me."

"It's not my fault I eat too much; my mom taught me to clean my plate."

"I'm having trouble meeting this deadline because the client keeps changing his mind. I'm miserable, and it's all his fault!"

"My girlfriend didn't call on time, and now it's too late to go to that movie I wanted to see. She's ruined my night!"

"My husband did not protect me from the bad decision I made at work."

"It's my boss's fault I did not get promoted."

"It's my child's fault."

"It's the teacher's fault my child is failing."

"It wasn't my fault that I wasn't prepared for the meeting. They never give enough notice."

"That wouldn't have happened if you had been better to me."

"How was I supposed to know the boss wanted the reports in two days? He should have told me."

"If it was so important, why didn't you remind me?"

"That's not my job."

Beginning a sentence with "It is your fault that I . . ." can ruin your life. Blaming ANTs make you a victim, and when you are a victim, you are powerless to change your behavior.

Less-Than ANTs. Less-Than ANTs are some of the most toxic ANTs to your self-esteem. Whenever you compare yourself to others in a negative way, these ANTs harass and attack you. They are involved in the epidemic rise of teenage depression and suicide, all exacerbated by social media. Many teens spend hours a day comparing their lives and the way they look to a false sense of others'. Parents can also put unrealistic expectations and pressure on their children to live up to those on the internet. Marcus's comment that "I am not as smart as the other kids" is a classic example of Less-Than thinking.

Less-Than ANTs are easy to identify because, like Marcus's statement, they usually start with the words "I am not . . ."

I am not good enough.
I am not a good enough mother/father.
I am not a good enough son/daughter.

I am not a good enough wife/husband.
I am not a good enough boss/employee.
I am not a good enough Christian.
I am not a good enough investor.
I am not smart enough.
I am not rich enough.
I am not tall enough.
I am not strong enough.
I am not pretty enough.
I am not funny enough.
I am not kind enough.

If you continually compete with and compare yourself to others, you'll have lower self-esteem, and you will be bitter. If you compete to be your best self, you will be better. The problem is often we are comparing our behind-the-scenes self with another person's highlight reel.

When I was a young psychiatrist, just out of my training, I noticed that people who looked like they had it all together (a great marriage, perfect children, career success, etc.) often would be in my office telling me about their troubles, such as a gambling addiction, extramarital affairs, and children who were stealing. I met parents with criminal records, a priest who no longer believed in God, and so on. It was such an important lesson. Few people are who they show to the outside world. I have had the honor of treating US senators, Oscar- and Emmy-winning actors, Hall of Fame athletes, Grammy-winning musicians, business leaders, and megachurch pastors. These wonderful people all had the same issues and insecurities as the rest of us.

When you allow the Less-Than ANTs to steal your happiness, you stop celebrating your wins, you come to resent the people you love, and you feel envious when others succeed.

"If-Only" and "I'll-Be-Happy-When" ANTs. I once heard Byron Katie tell an audience, "Whenever you argue with reality, welcome to hell." I have shared that line many times with my patients. Spending time in regret for things in the past you cannot change leads only to pain and ongoing frustration. Regret manifests itself in "If only . . ." thinking patterns for what occurred and "I'll be happy when . . ." for regrets in the present you hope will change in the future. Each of these phrases ensures self-defeating thoughts because they take you out of the present moment. The other side of regret is unhappiness with the present, hoping for a different future. In Marcus's case, he thought all of his problems could have been avoided if he hadn't changed schools. Other examples of these happiness-stealing ANTs include:

> *If only I had sold my stocks before the economy tanked.*
> *If only my parents had been rich.*
> *If only I were taller/skinnier/prettier.*
> *If only I had stayed in school.*
> *If only I hadn't made that mistake.*
> *If only I had stopped drinking earlier.*
> *I'll be happier when I retire.*
> *I'll be happier when he/she agrees to marry me.*
> *I'll be happier when our divorce is finalized.*
> *I'll be happier when I have children.*
> *I'll be happier when the children are grown and out of my hair.*
> *I'll be happier when I graduate from college.*
> *I'll be happier when I land that promotion.*
> *I'll be happier when I lose 10 pounds.*

Left unchecked, these ANTs will ruin your relationships, your self-esteem, and eventually, your life.

The good news is, you can learn to eliminate your ANTs and replace them with more helpful thoughts that give you a more accurate, fair assessment of any situation. I'm not talking about positive thinking that ignores reality. I'm talking about accurate, honest thinking. We'll talk more about how to do this in the next chapter, but rest assured, with a bit of practice, you can learn how to squash your ANTs and lead a happier, healthier life!

CHAPTER 2

YOU ARE WHAT YOU THINK

As you think, so you feel,
As you feel, so you do, and
As you do, so you have.

JOSEPH McCLENDON III,
author of *Get Happy Now!*

WHEN I WAS A YOUNG PSYCHIATRIST, I used a technique called biofeedback to help understand and treat my patients. Biofeedback uses instruments to measure hand temperature, sweat gland activity, muscle tension, breathing rate, heart rate, and brain wave patterns. If we know how your body reacts to stress, we can teach you to soothe it. Your conscious and unconscious brain expresses its aspirations, worries, fears, stress, love, joy, hatred, and happiness through your body's reactions. Knowing this, I developed a word association test to see how my patients'

33

bodies respond to certain words and concepts. I hook them up to biofeedback equipment as I would to a lie detector machine and then ask them to think about certain words. Some of the words are innocuous, such as *telephone*, *book*, or *paper clip*, and other words have more emotional meanings, such as *mother*, *father*, *siblings*, *job*, *children*, and *spouse*.

Most people have only small physiological reactions to innocuous words but much larger reactions to emotionally loaded words. For example, if I say *baseball* or *train*, there is usually little movement in the biofeedback equipment, unless a person loves a baseball team or collects model trains. However, when I say words like *mother* or *father*, I usually see a significant change. If *mother* is a positive concept in the person's life, like mine is for me, the changes move in a positive direction: heart and breathing rates slow, muscles become more relaxed, hands become warmer and drier. If *mother* is associated with painful or stressful memories, the change usually goes in a stressful direction: heart and breathing rates escalate, muscles become tense, hands become colder, and sweat gland activity increases.

Through biofeedback, I've learned that your brain is always listening and responding to every thought you have, especially the stressful and positive ones. The thousands of thoughts you have every day are based on myriad factors, including past experiences, sensory input, dreams, what you had for dinner last night, and the health of your gut bacteria. Negative thoughts cause your brain to immediately release chemicals that affect every cell in your body, making you feel bad; while the opposite is also true—positive, happy, hopeful thoughts release chemicals that make you feel good. Your thought patterns can also have long-term effects. Repetitive negative thinking may promote the buildup of the harmful deposits seen in the brains of people with Alzheimer's disease and may increase the risk of dementia, according to a 2020 brain imaging study in *Alzheimer's & Dementia*.[1]

Thoughts are also automatic. They just happen. And just because you have a thought has nothing to do with whether it is true. Thoughts lie. They lie a lot, and it is your uninvestigated or unquestioned thoughts that steal your

Just because you have a thought has nothing to do with whether it is true.

happiness. If you do not question or correct your erroneous thoughts, you believe them, and you act as if they are 100 percent true. For example, if I thought, *My wife never listens to me*, it would make me feel sad and lonely, and eventually, a little angry. If I never questioned the negative thought, even though it isn't true, I would act as if it were true and give myself permission to be irritable with her, making it less likely she would ever *want* to listen to me. Allowing yourself to believe every thought you have is the prescription for anxiety disorders, depression, relationship problems, and chronic illness. You must protect yourself from the negative thoughts that are trying to steal your happiness. And to do that, you need to learn how to squash your ANTs (automatic negative thoughts).

But first, let's take a brief tour of your brain, so you can better understand how ANTs impact not only your emotional health, but your physical and spiritual health as well.

INSIDE VIEW OF THE BRAIN

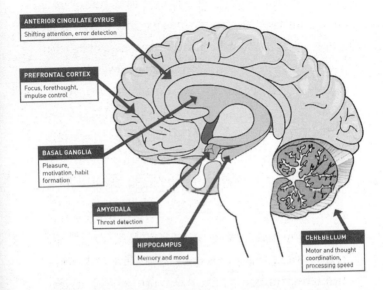

ANTERIOR CINGULATE GYRUS
Shifting attention, error detection

PREFRONTAL CORTEX
Focus, forethought, impulse control

BASAL GANGLIA
Pleasure, motivation, habit formation

AMYGDALA
Threat detection

HIPPOCAMPUS
Memory and mood

CEREBELLUM
Motor and thought coordination, processing speed

Your Brain: A Very Brief Primer

As we embark on this journey together, it's important to briefly get acquainted with six brain systems involved in running your life. Obviously, your brain is complicated and involves many different structures, but these are particularly important as they work in concert to create your moods, anxieties, memory, and behavior.

Prefrontal cortex (PFC): Found in the front third of the brain, the PFC plays a major role in executive functions (like the boss at work), such as focus, forethought, judgment, planning, decision making, and impulse control. When it is low in activity from head trauma, toxins, attention deficit hyperactivity disorder (ADHD), or other causes, people tend to struggle with attention, distractibility, disorganization, procrastination, and impulsive behavior. It is like the boss went on vacation.

Anterior cingulate gyrus (ACG): Found deep within the frontal lobes, it is involved with shifting attention and error detection. When the ACG is overactive, people tend to struggle with getting stuck on negative thoughts or behaviors, worrying, being oppositional or argumentative, or seeing too many errors in themselves or others.

Amygdala (AMY): This almond-shaped structure is found underneath the temples and behind the eyes; there is one on each side of the brain. They are involved in emotion, threat detection, and aggression. They tend to be overactive in people who have past emotional trauma, are hypervigilant (always watching for something bad to happen), and are socially anxious. When the AMY are underactive, people tend to have less fear, like the rock climber in *Free Solo*, and be risk-takers.

Hippocampus (HC): Greek for "seahorse" (*hippo*—horse; *kampos*—sea monster), your two hippocampi (plural) are about the size of your thumbs and found deep in the brain on the inside of your left and right temporal lobes, just behind the amygdala. They are part of your emotional brain and help you feel happy or sad and are central to memory. They retain new information and store it for up to several weeks; if it is reinforced, you keep it longer. If the hippocampi are damaged, you cannot store new information. In the movie *50 First Dates*, Lucy, Drew Barrymore's character, had a severe car accident that damaged her left and right hippocampi. After she falls asleep, memories of the prior day are wiped out. Memory problems are associated with low activity in the HC, and it is one of the first areas of the brain that dies in Alzheimer's disease. The HC also can produce up to 700 new stem cells a day if put in a nourishing environment (think good nutrition, omega-3 fatty acids, oxygen levels, blood flow, and mental stimulation).[2]

Basal ganglia (BG): These large structures deep in the brain are involved in habit formation. The BG also contain the nucleus accumbens (NA), which is part of your reward system (motivates you to go toward pleasure and away from pain), and is exquisitely responsive to the feel-good neurotransmitter dopamine, involved in addictions. The NA is involved with cravings. If it is underactive, people tend to feel flat and depressed, and they are more vulnerable to addiction and to craving the substances that activate it, such as drugs, alcohol, sex, or high-calorie sugary foods.

Cerebellum (CB): Latin for "little brain," it is located at the back, bottom portion of the brain. It is only 10 percent of the brain's volume, yet it contains half of the brain's neurons or cells. It is involved in coordination, processing speed, cognitive processing, and language.

The Four Circles of Health and Illness

These biological systems of the brain represent one of four circles of overall physical and mental health, which I think about whenever I evaluate or treat any patient. I first wrote about them in my book *Change Your Brain, Change Your Life*.[3] Here's a brief description of each of those four circles:

Biological: How the physical aspects of your brain and body function. One of the major principles of my work is that if you want to keep the physical functioning of your brain healthy or rescue it if it is headed for trouble, you have to prevent or treat the 11 major risk factors that steal your mind. My team created the mnemonic BRIGHT MINDS to summarize them: blood flow, retirement/aging, inflammation, genetics, head trauma, toxins, mental health (abnormal electrical activity), immunity and infections (relevant after a pandemic), neurohormones, diabesity (a combination of being overweight and having high blood sugar), and sleep disturbances.[4] The biological circle also encompasses diet and exercise.

Psychological: How you think and talk to yourself, as well as self-concept, body image, emotional trauma, upbringing, and significant life events. ANTs influence your psychological health by saying whether you are enough—good enough, smart enough, pretty enough, strong enough, rich enough, and so on. When you've squashed your ANTs and believe that you are enough, you will be happier and more confident. When you feel less than enough, your brain can give in to sadness, anxiety, and failure.

Social: The quality of your relationships and any current life stresses. When you have solid relationships, a healthy family, a role or career you enjoy, and financial stability, your brain tends to do much better than when any of these areas are troubled. Your ANTs can take over when difficult life situations, such as an illness, relationship breakup or divorce, layoff, or death of a loved one, elevate stress hormone levels. When this circle is unhealthy, you are more vulnerable to illnesses, as well as depression, anxiety disorders, and more.

Spiritual: Your connection to God, the planet, and past and future generations; and your deepest sense of meaning and purpose. You are more than just your brain cells, thoughts, and connections. I believe we are all created with divine purpose. When your brain listens to ANTs, it's easy to forget that your life matters and that you have a role and a calling to fulfill.

When any one circle is unhealthy, your brain is more likely to listen to your ANTs and let them take control. Now, let's talk about how to squash those ANTs and regain control of your brain, your health, and your life!

Killing Your ANTs

My ANT killing process is based on the work of two mentors: psychiatrist Aaron Beck, who pioneered a school of psychotherapy called cognitive behavioral therapy (CBT), which is an effective treatment for anxiety disorders, depression, relationship problems, and even obesity; and Byron Katie, a teacher and author who developed the five questions we'll discuss later in appendix A to kill ANTs.

How you feel is often related to the quality of your thoughts. If they are mostly negative, you will feel mostly negative; if they are mostly positive, you will feel mostly positive. ANTs link, stack, and multiply with other ANTs to attack you. For instance, the ANTs grow stronger and increase in number before bed, when you get less sleep, when your blood sugar is low, in winter, right before a woman's menstrual cycle, when you're under stress, and when you lose someone you love.

Every time you have a thought, your brain releases chemicals.

That's how your brain works. You have a thought, your brain releases chemicals, electrical transmissions travel throughout your brain, and you become aware of what you're thinking. Thoughts are real, and they have a powerful impact on how you feel and behave. Just as a muscle that's exercised becomes stronger, repeatedly thinking the same thoughts makes them stronger too.

Every time you have an angry, unkind, hopeless, helpless, worthless, sad, or irritating thought, such as *I'm stupid*, your brain releases chemicals that make you feel bad. In this way, your body reacts to every negative thought you have. Marcus was exercising his brain to feel depression, sadness, and failure. I asked him to think about the last time he was mad. How did his body feel? When most people are angry, their muscles become tense, their hearts beat faster, their hands start to sweat, and they may even begin to feel a little dizzy. Marcus told me he got dizzy and sweaty and felt confused and stupid.

Similarly, every time you have a happy, hopeful, kind, optimistic, positive thought, your brain releases chemicals that make you feel good. I asked Marcus to think about the last time he had a happy thought. How did he feel inside his body? When most people are happy, their muscles relax, their hearts beat more slowly, their hands become dry, and they breathe more evenly. Marcus told me about an outing with his father, where they went fishing and had a great time. When he thought about it, he said he felt peaceful and happy. He didn't feel stupid.

Thoughts are powerful, and your body reacts to every single one you have.

Thoughts can make your mind and body feel good, or they can make you feel bad. Every cell in your body is affected by every thought you have. We know this from polygraph, or lie detector, tests. During a polygraph, a person is connected to instruments that measure:

- hand temperature
- heart rate
- blood pressure
- breathing rate
- muscle tension
- sweat gland activity

The tester then asks questions, such as "Did you do that misdeed?" Almost immediately, the tested person's body reacts to every thought they have, whether they say anything or not. If the person did it and worries they'll be found out, their body is likely to have a stress response and react in the following ways:

- hand temperature drops
- heart rate speeds up
- blood pressure increases

- breathing rate increases, but breaths are more shallow
- muscle tension increases
- sweat gland activity increases

The opposite is also true. If they did not do the deed, their body will experience a relaxation response and react in the following ways:

- hand temperature increases
- heart rate slows
- blood pressure decreases
- breathing rate decreases and breaths become deeper
- muscle tension decreases
- sweat gland activity decreases

Again, your body reacts almost immediately to what you think—and not just when you're asked about telling the truth. Your body reacts to every thought you have, whether it is about work, friends, family, or anything else. This is why when people become upset, they often develop physical symptoms, such as headaches, stomachaches, or diarrhea, or they become more susceptible to illness. Imagine what was happening in Marcus's young body as his mind was flooded with negative thoughts.

As I mentioned at the start of this chapter, Amen Clinics uses biofeedback equipment to measure the same physiological responses as polygraphs: hand temperature, heart rate, breathing rate, muscle tension, and sweat gland activity. I hooked up Marcus to our equipment. When I asked him about baseball (a sport he loved), his baby sister, and his friends, his body showed an immediate relaxation response. Yet when I asked him about school, feeling stupid, or his history teacher (with whom he was having a particularly hard time), his hands immediately got colder, his heart rate and muscle tension increased, his breathing rate became disorganized, and his hands started to sweat more. Marcus and his mother were amazed to see the evidence of how his body responded to every thought he had.

I taught Marcus to think of his body as an "ecosystem" that contains everything in the environment, such as air, water, land, cars, people, animals, vegetation, houses, landfills, and more.

A negative thought was like pollution to his whole system. Just as pollution in Los Angeles or Beijing affects everyone who goes outdoors, negative thoughts pollute your mind and your body.

Your thoughts are hardwired to be negative.

In generations past, negative thoughts protected us from early death or becoming supper for powerful animals. From our earliest times on earth, being aware of and avoiding danger was crucial to survival. Unfortunately, even when the world became safer, negativity bias remained in our brains. Researchers have demonstrated that negative experiences have a greater impact on the brain than positive ones.[5] People pay more attention to negative than to positive news, which is why news outlets typically lead broadcasts with floods, murders, political disasters, and all forms of mayhem. According to research from the content marketing website Outbrain.com, in two periods of 2012 the average click-through rate on headlines with negative adjectives was an astounding 63 percent higher than for headlines with positive ones.[6] A negative perspective is more contagious than a positive one, which may be why political campaigns typically go negative at the end. Even our language is not exempt: 62 percent of the words in the English dictionary connote negative emotions, while 32 percent express positive ones.[7]

Psychologist and author Rick Hanson has written that the brain is wired for negativity bias. Bad news is quickly stored in the brain to keep us safe, but positive experiences have to be held in consciousness for more than 12 seconds before they stay with us. "The brain is like Velcro for negative experiences but Teflon for positive ones," Hanson wrote.[8] Psychologist Mihaly Csikszentmihalyi, author of *Flow: The Psychology of Optimal Experience*, suggested that without other thoughts to occupy us, our brains will always return to worry. The only way to escape this is to focus on what will bring "flow"—activities that increase our sense of purpose and achievement.

Negative emotions "trump" positive emotions, which is why it is critical to discipline our natural tendency toward the negative and amplify more helpful thoughts and emotions. I taught Marcus that his negative thought pattern was common but not helpful.

Thoughts are automatic and often lie.

Thoughts are based on complex chemical reactions in the brain; memories from the past; the quality of our sleep, hormones, and blood sugar; and many other factors. They are automatic, reflexive, random, and overwhelmingly negative. Plus, they are often erroneous. Unless disciplined and bridled, they will lie to you and wreak havoc in your life. Marcus thought he was stupid. He told himself so multiple times a day because he had trouble staying focused and didn't perform well on tests. Yet when we tested him, his IQ was 135—in the top one percent of all people. I told him it was critical to question every stupid thought that went through his head.

It's important to examine your thoughts to see if they are true and if they are helping you or hurting you. Unfortunately, if you never challenge your thoughts, you will simply believe them and then act out of that erroneous belief.

By repeatedly allowing his undisciplined thoughts to invade his mind, telling himself he was stupid, a failure, and a terrible person who hated school and was hated by his teachers, Marcus was more likely to behave in ways that would make those terrible things happen. I told him that his brain makes happen what it sees, which is why it is critical to get control over your thoughts.

Seven Strategies to Master Your Mind

It is possible to learn how to listen to your thoughts and redirect them so that you feel happier and more positive. Here are seven strategies that will help you put what I have just discussed into practice.

Strategy #1: Eliminate ANTs as they attack.
Get a journal or use the notes app on your phone, and whenever you feel sad, mad, nervous, or out of control,

1. Write down your automatic negative thoughts (ANTs).

2. Identify the ANT species. (It may be more than one.)

3. Ask yourself if you are 100 percent sure the thought is true.

Shining a beam of truth on the ANTs causes them to disintegrate. Here are six examples from my patients:

1. **FROM A WOMAN WHO WAS RAPED, WHO CAME TO SEE ME FOR ANXIETY AND DEPRESSION:**

ANT: *I am fractured.*

ANT species: She listed it as an All-or-Nothing and Labeling ANT.

Is it true? "It is not true," she wrote. "I am a good person who was attacked. I can overcome it to become whole." Talking back to the thought takes away its power.

2. **FROM A FATHER WHOSE ADULT SON WAS A DRUG ADDICT:**

ANT: *I am not a good father.*

ANT species: He listed it as an All-or-Nothing and Guilt-Beating ANT.

Is it true? "It is not true," he wrote. "I was present and loving. Addiction runs in our family, but ultimately it was my son's choice to engage in behaviors where he lost control. I will be there to support him as I can, but I cannot control his life."

3. **FROM A WOMAN WHOSE SON WAS MURDERED:**

ANT: *I am evil for wanting his murderer to be punished.*

ANT species: She listed it as a Labeling ANT.

Is it true? "It is not true," she wrote. "I am a good person with a loving heart. I miss my son so much and have hope I will see him again in heaven."

4. **FROM A WOMAN HAVING MARITAL PROBLEMS, WHO FELT HERSELF BECOMING MORE CLINGY AND DESPERATE:**

ANT: *My husband will leave me and I will be all alone.*

ANT species: She listed it as a Fortune-Telling ANT.

Is it true? She wrote, "I don't know if it is true, but if I keep acting anxious and desperate, he *will* leave me. I need to be strong no matter what happens."

5. **FROM A MAN WHO WAS FIRED FROM WORK BECAUSE OF HIS TEMPER:**

ANT: *I am a bad person and will never find another job. My family will be destitute.*

ANT species: He listed it as a Labeling and Fortune-Telling ANT.

Is it true? "I need to understand and fix my temper," he told me. "I am a good person and will work to find another job to care for my family and myself."

6. **FROM A YOUNG ADULT WHO WAS STRUGGLING IN COLLEGE:**

ANT: *I'll never be as good as my friends.*

ANT species: He listed it as an All-or-Nothing ANT.

Is it true? He told me, "I am better than

my friends at some things and not at others. I need to stop being so hard on myself."

Confronting ANTs with truth is a powerful tool. Several months after Marcus learned to eliminate the ANTs, his anxiety and depression were remarkably reduced and his school performance improved. He went on to graduate from college with honors and eventually from law school. Don't believe every stupid thought you have.

Strategy #2: Stop monkey mind by paying attention to it.

We all deal with disjointed thoughts at times, but one of the best ways to stop the monkeys from ruining your mind with all their distractions is to start paying attention to them. When you ignore your inner life, like attention-starved children the monkeys start to misbehave, torture you, belittle you, and wreak all sorts of havoc. However, when you start noticing your thoughts, evaluating them, or even being amused by them, they loosen their control over your emotional life.

Taking time to reflect and direct your inner life can help you train the monkeys to work for you, rather than threaten your sanity. Meditation is a wonderful way to get control of your mind. Research has shown that meditation can slow your heart rate; lower your blood pressure; increase your circulation; aid your digestion; strengthen your immune system; improve your cognition, focus, and memory; and decrease your brain aging, addictions, anxiety, depression, and irritability.[9] You might consider trying loving-kindness meditation, in which you direct thoughts of love, compassion, and goodwill toward yourself, those close to you, and others with whom you have strained relationships. Devoting a few minutes each day to a meditation practice, whether by meditating on a Scripture passage or doing loving-kindness meditation, will help you quiet your mind.

Strategy #3: Start every day with the phrase "Today is going to be a great day."

As soon as you awaken or your feet hit the floor in the morning, say these words out loud. Since your mind is prone to negativity, it will find stress in the upcoming day unless you train and discipline it. When you direct your thoughts to "Today is going to be a great day," your brain will help you uncover the reasons why it will be so. When I'm on a tour for public television, for example, and I wake up in a different city every morning, my brain could anticipate everything that could go wrong, including the hassles of travel, causing me to feel lousy. Instead, when I say, "Today is going to be a great day," I think of all the wonderful people I'll meet or lives that may be changed by our work, and I enjoy the journey.

You have a choice in where you direct your attention, even in times of loss. This simple strategy can make a powerfully positive difference in your life.

Strategy #4: Record your moods and look for ways to increase gratitude.

Business professionals frequently say, "You cannot change what you do not measure." That's why it's smart to keep a daily journal to record and measure the feeling(s) you want to decrease, such as anxiety, fear, sadness, anger, or grief, or that you want to increase, such as joy, happiness, or another emotion. Write down a feeling and evaluate it on a scale from 1 to 10, where 1 is "awful" and 10 is "great." Whenever you have a difficult day or several days, you can look at your journal and try to spot trends, such as certain days of the week and times of the day, the time of your menstrual cycle, whether you have eaten or not, and more.

One of the early lessons I learned as a psychiatrist was that I could make nearly anyone cry or feel upset by the questions I asked. If I asked people to think about their worst memories—the times they failed, the incidents where they were most embarrassed, or the day they lost someone they loved—within seconds they would feel bad. But the opposite was also true. If I asked them to think about their happiest moments—the times they succeeded or their experiences of falling in love—they generally started to smile. Here are six quick journaling exercises to help you change your focus.

1. **Write out three things for which you are grateful.** Gratitude helps direct your attention toward positive feelings and away from negative ones. Dr. Hans Selye, considered one of the pioneers of stress research, wrote, "Nothing erases unpleasant thoughts more effectively than conscious concentration on pleasant ones."[10] If I could bottle gratitude, I would. The benefits far outweigh almost all of the medications I prescribe, without any side effects. A wealth of research suggests that a daily practice of gratitude, which can be as simple as writing down several things we're grateful for every day, can improve our emotions, health, relationships, personalities, and careers. From a wonderful blog post by Amit Amin[11] at the Happier Human and Courtney Ackerman at Positive Psychology Program,[12] research suggests that gratitude can enhance

   - Happiness
   - Well-being
   - Mood
   - Self-esteem
   - Resilience

- Sense of spirituality
- Impulse to give
- Optimism
- Reduction in materialism
- Reduction in self-centeredness
- Recovery from substance misuse
- Resistance to stress
- Resistance to envy
- Friendships
- Love relationships
- Career
- Networking ability
- Productivity
- Goal achievement
- Reduction in turnover
- Decision-making
- Physical health, including:
  - Physical appearance
  - Better sleep
  - Fewer physical symptoms
  - More time exercising
  - Less physical pain

- Lower blood pressure in people who were hypertensive
- Recovery from coronary events
- Vitality and energy
- Longevity[13]

Focusing on gratitude has been found to increase the activity of the parasympathetic nervous system and decrease inflammatory markers;[14] improve depression, stress, and happiness;[15] reduce stress among caregivers;[16] and, among the elderly, significantly decrease state anxiety and depression as well as increase specific memories, life satisfaction, and subjective happiness.[17]

When you make a habit of bringing your attention to the things you're grateful for, you enhance how your brain works. In times of stress, take a minute to write down three things—big or small—that you're grateful for. You might find you have trouble stopping at three.

2. **Write a letter.** Expressing your appreciation in writing to someone will benefit both them

and you Martin Seligman, PhD, considered the father of positive psychology, and his team at the University of Pennsylvania developed the gratitude letter exercise. (See pages 100–101 for more details.) Research has shown that this practice significantly increases life satisfaction scores and happiness and decreases symptoms of depression.[18]

3. **Express your appreciation.** To enhance gratitude, add appreciation, which is gratitude that is outwardly expressed and builds bridges between people. Expressing support and appreciation to others has been shown to decrease the stress response in the brain much more powerfully than receiving support.[19] *It is better for your brain to give than to receive.* To supercharge joyful thinking, get in the habit of writing down the name of one person whom you appreciate and why; then share your feelings with that person with a quick email, text, or call. Do this once a week and try not to repeat anyone for two months. This exercise will help you build many bridges of goodwill.

4. **Count your blessings.** You can boost your good feelings if you count your blessings instead of sheep at night. In a study of 221 teenagers, the group that focused on counting their blessings reported increases in gratitude, optimism, and life satisfaction and decreases in negative feelings.[20] At bedtime, write down as many good things in your life as you can think of in three minutes.

5. **Note what went well.** Another exercise that has been shown to quickly increase your level of well-being is called "What Went Well." Research has shown that people who did this exercise were happier and less depressed at one-month and six-month follow-ups than at the study's outset.[21] Right before bed, write down three things that went well that day; then ask yourself, "Why did this happen?" This simple exercise has been found to help people in stressful jobs develop more positive emotions.[22]

6. **Focus on your accomplishments.** I once treated a very successful businesswoman who made millions of dollars. She was struggling

with anxiety and depression, and she felt that she was a failure and her life was worthless. She repeatedly focused on one incident where a reporter, who as far as I could tell accomplished little in his life except trashing successful people, had harshly criticized her in a magazine article. She played the article over and over in her mind. She had an obsessive pattern in her brain, where she tended to get stuck on negative thoughts and behaviors.

Her first homework assignment was to write out her accomplishments in as much detail as she liked. At her next session she brought eight pages full of accomplishments, including employing 500 people, doing charity work, and maintaining strong relationships. The exercise made her feel great and quickly changed her focus.

Write down the highest and most positive moments of your life. If you can find one moment, odds are you can find two. If you can find two, you can likely find four, and so on. By bringing your attention to your successes, you are much more likely to feel better fast.

Strategy #5: Create optimism with a dose of reality to build resilience fast.

Dr. Seligman developed a concept known as learned helplessness that has had a powerful influence over my career.[23] He found that when dogs, rats, mice, and even cockroaches experienced painful shocks over which they had no control, eventually they would just accept the pain without attempting to escape. Humans, he discovered, do the same thing. In a series of experiments, his research team randomly divided subjects into three groups: those who were exposed to a loud noise they could stop by pushing a button; those who heard the irritating noise but couldn't turn it off; and a control group who heard nothing at all. The following day the subjects faced a new research task that again involved painful sounds. To turn it off, all they had to do was move their hands about 12 inches. The people in the first and third groups figured this out quickly and were able to turn off the noise. But most of the people in the second group did nothing at all. Expecting failure, they didn't even try to escape the irritating noise. They had learned to be helpless.

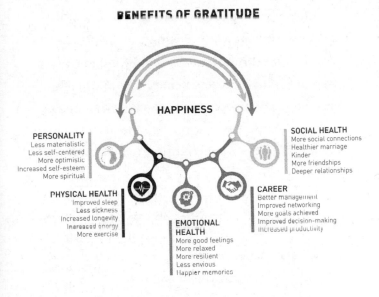

BENEFITS OF GRATITUDE

HAPPINESS

PERSONALITY
Less materialistic
Less self-centered
More optimistic
Increased self-esteem
More spiritual

SOCIAL HEALTH
More social connections
Healthier marriage
Kinder
More friendships
Deeper relationships

PHYSICAL HEALTH
Improved sleep
Less sickness
Increased longevity
Increased energy
More exercise

EMOTIONAL HEALTH
More good feelings
More relaxed
More resilient
Less envious
Happier memories

CAREER
Better management
Improved networking
More goals achieved
Improved decision-making
Increased productivity

Yet—and this is where it gets exciting—about one-third of the people in group two, who had been unable to escape the pain, never became helpless. Why? The answer turned out to be optimism. Dr. Seligman's team discovered that people who do not give up interpret the pain and setbacks as

- *temporary* as opposed to permanent;
- *limited* instead of pervasive; and
- *changeable* instead of out of their control.

Optimists would say things like "It will go away quickly; it's just this one situation, and I can do something about it." Dr. Seligman's team came to believe that teaching optimism could help inoculate people against anxiety, depression, post-traumatic stress disorder, and relationship problems. Here are some of his main ideas:

1. *Listen to yourself and others to see how things are explained.* Are the people powerful or victims? Do they have control or no control? Are hardships permanent or temporary? *Pessimists* describe *bad* things as permanent and pervasive and *good* things as temporary, while *optimists* describe things in just the reverse: the bad as temporary and the *good* as permanent and pervasive.

2. *Change your language and feelings around the situations you face.* You can stop being a victim, take control wherever possible, and understand that hardships are usually temporary.

3. *Allow mistakes to be learning experiences, rather than a final judgment on your self-worth.* Everyone makes mistakes; it's how you

respond to them that determines how quickly you recover. Accepting a mistake and looking for the lesson you can take away from it will help you get over it and move on.

Pessimism and Optimism Are Habits of Thinking

PESSIMISTS (FEEL HELPLESS)	OPTIMISTS (FEEL HOPEFUL)
See problems as permanent	See problems as temporary
See problems as pervasive	See problems as limited
See no personal control	See personal control or influence
See failure as a statement about self	See failure as a lesson
Have low self-efficacy	Feel self-confident
Focus on problems	Are forward thinking
Tend to be hopeless	Tend to be hopeful
Tend to give up	Tend to stick with difficult things
Are less proactive with health	Are more proactive with health

Hold grudges	Forgive more easily
Focus on worries and negativity	Are less likely to dwell on the negative
Feel more stressed	Feel less stressed
Are more likely to have insomnia	Are more likely to sleep better
See glass as half-empty	See glass as half-full
Are more withholding	Are more altruistic

Strive to take control of your life, be forward thinking, and see possibilities. A huge study involving more than 97,000 people found that those who were optimistic had significantly lower heart disease than those who were pessimistic.[24] Women who scored highly on "cynical hostility" were also more likely to develop coronary heart disease. Optimism is also associated with a higher quality of life,[25] a lower incidence of stroke,[26] improved immune system function,[27] better pain tolerance,[28] and longer survival in lung cancer patients.[29]

Yet as we've seen, blind optimism can lead to early death. The Longevity Project from

Stanford University found that people who were mindlessly optimistic died the earliest from accidents and preventable illnesses.[30] Being sleep-deprived led to increased optimism and poorer life choices.[31] College students who were too optimistic had more binge-drinking behavior,[32] and compulsive gamblers were often rated as too optimistic.[33] The bottom line: It is always best to balance optimism with planning for and preventing future trouble. Being optimistic about eating a third bowl of ice cream with caramel sauce will lead to early death, no matter how much you wish it wouldn't.

Strategy #6: Change the B stuff.

We are not controlled by events or people, but by our perceptions of them.

I once heard the following story: At the turn of the century a shoe company sent a representative to Africa. He wired back, "I'm coming home. No one wears shoes here." Another company sent their representative, who sold thousands of shoes. He wired back to his company, "Business is fantastic. No one has ever heard of shoes here." The two representatives perceived the same situation from markedly different perspectives, and they obtained dramatically different results.

Perception is the way we, as individuals, interpret ourselves and the world around us. Our five senses take in the world, but perception occurs as our brains process the incoming information through our "feeling filters." When our filters feel good, we translate information in a positive way. When our filters are angry or hostile, we perceive the world as negative toward us. Our perceptions of the outside world are based on our inner worlds. When we're feeling tired, for example, we're much more likely to be irritated by a child's behavior that usually doesn't bother us.

Our view of a situation has a greater impact on our lives than the situation itself. Noted psychiatrist Richard Gardner said that the world is like a Rorschach test, where a person is asked to describe what he or she sees in 10 inkblots that mean absolutely nothing. What we see in the inkblot is based on our inner view of the world; our perceptions bear witness to our state of mind. As we think, so do we perceive. Therefore, in reality, we need not seek to change the outside world but rather to change our inner worlds. I teach all of my patients the *A-B-C* model:

A is the actual event,
B is how we interpret or perceive the event,
and
C is how we react to the event.

Other people or events (*A*) can't make us do anything. It is our interpretation or perception (*B*) that causes our behavior (*C*). Consider, for instance, the time I yawned during a therapy session with a patient. He asked if I found him boring. I replied that it was important that he asked. I had been up most of the previous night with an emergency and was tired, but I found what he was saying very interesting. My yawning was *A*, his interpretation that I was bored was *B*, and his asking me about it was *C*. I was glad he asked about my yawn because some patients' *C* would have been to leave the therapy session with a negative feeling. When we can allow ourselves to look at the alternatives and challenge our initial negative perceptions, we've traveled a long way toward emotional health.

Questioning the *B* stuff is so important. It can make the difference between a meaningful life and death. Think about the two New Testament stories of Judas and Peter, two of Jesus' disciples, betraying Jesus on the night he was arrested (see Matthew 26:69–27:10). Judas accepted money to identify Jesus to the Temple guards, who arrested him. Later that night Peter denied three times that he even knew Jesus. *A* was betrayal. *B* was their interpretation of the betrayal: Judas felt he had committed an unforgivable sin; Peter was ashamed and wept. *C* was each of their reactions: Judas returned the 30 pieces of silver and then hanged himself, while Peter asked for and was given forgiveness and later became a central figure in starting the Christian church. If we don't question our perceptions, they can take us to places we don't want to go.

Strategy #7: Watch the Disney movie Pollyanna. One of my favorite movies of all time is the Disney movie *Pollyanna*, based on the 1913 book of the same name by Eleanor Porter. After her missionary parents died, Pollyanna came to live with her aunt Polly and was able to help turn a divided small town with many negative people into a positive community. She introduced them to "the glad game," which involved looking for things to be glad about in any situation. Her father had taught her this game once when she was very disappointed. She had always wanted a doll, but her parents never had enough money to buy one for her. When her father asked his missionary sponsors to send a secondhand doll, by mistake they sent Pollyanna a pair of crutches. *How can I be glad about crutches?* she wondered. Then she decided she could be glad because she didn't need to use them. This simple game changed the attitudes and lives of many people in the movie. Pollyanna even told the minister what her father had taught her: The Bible had 800 "glad passages," and if God mentioned being glad that many times, it must be because he wants us to think that way.

Focusing on the negative in situations will make you feel bad. Playing the glad game, or looking for the positive, will help you feel better. This movie is worth the 134-minute investment.

It's no exaggeration to say that developing accurate, honest, and disciplined thinking can change your life. If you get rid of the ANTs, practice gratitude, manage your perceptions, and follow these other strategies, you'll see a decrease in worry, anxiety, anger, and negativity and be on your way to feeling better fast.

Love—Your Secret Weapon

When Jesus told us to love each other as ourselves, he was giving us good health advice. Research suggests that whenever you feel down, anxious, or angry, it is best to get outside yourself to change your state of mind. In a new study, people who wrote about gratitude activated a part of their brains involved in happiness and altruism.[34]

That said, if you want to feel better, go to the aid of someone who needs help. According to a *New York Times* story, in the 1970s, former First Lady Barbara Bush became so depressed that she sometimes stopped her car on the side of the road for fear that she might deliberately crash the vehicle into a tree or an oncoming car. Mrs.

Bush did not seek psychiatric help or medication for her depression, which she blamed on the hormonal changes of menopause and the stress of her husband's job as CIA director. Instead, she said she treated her depression by immersing herself in volunteer work and getting outside herself to help others.[35]

Being loving to strangers—or even to people you know—has the added benefit of making you feel happier, according to two studies. In one study, 86 participants were asked about their life satisfaction and then divided into three groups. The first group was told to do an act of kindness every day for 10 days; the second group was told to do something new every day for 10 days; and the third group was given no instruction. When the 10 days had passed, the groups were retested on life satisfaction. Levels of happiness increased significantly and nearly equally among participants in the groups that had performed acts of kindness or novel activities, while happiness didn't change at all in the group that did neither.[36] Doing something for others for 10 days, especially if you vary the good deeds, is an

Being loving to strangers—or even to people you know—has the added benefit of making you feel happier.

effective way to make yourself feel better, the study suggests.

In another study, participants were divided into two groups and asked to recall either the last time they had spent either $20 or $100 on themselves or the last time they had spent the same amount on someone else. After completing a scale measuring their levels of happiness, all of the participants were provided with a small sum of money and given the option of spending the money on themselves or on another person. The researchers found that study subjects were happier when they were asked to recall a time when they had purchased something for someone else, no matter the price of the gift. What's more, the happier they felt about being generous in the past, the greater the likelihood that they would spend money on someone besides themselves.[37] As the Bible states, "It is more blessed to give than to receive" (Acts 20:35). Finally, research shows the happiest people are outward facing, focusing more on the people they serve than on themselves.[38]

Even though the prayer attributed to St. Francis of Assisi was likely not written by him, it still provides a research-based guide to happiness. The next time you feel down, consider repeating it or any other similar prayer or meditation, such as the loving-kindness meditation.

PEACE PRAYER OF SAINT FRANCIS

Lord, make me an instrument of your peace:
where there is hatred, let me sow love;
where there is injury, pardon;
where there is doubt, faith;
where there is despair, hope;
where there is darkness, light;
where there is sadness, joy.

O divine Master, grant that I may not
*   so much seek*
to be consoled as to console,
to be understood as to understand,
to be loved as to love.
For it is in giving that we receive,
it is in pardoning that we are pardoned,

*and it is in dying that we are born to
 eternal life.*
Amen.

By consciously bringing your attention to what you are grateful for, the people who bring you joy, and your own successes, you'll see a decrease in worry, anxiety, anger, and negativity and be on your way to feeling better fast.

CHAPTER 3

THE POWER OF POSITIVITY

"When you appreciate the good, the good appreciates."

TAL BEN-SHAHAR, author of *Choose the Life
You Want: The Mindful Way to Happiness*

I'LL NEVER FORGET THE MORNING of May 5, 2020, a Tuesday. I was in my bathroom, brushing my teeth and getting ready for a day that would begin with me driving my 90-year-old father, Louis Amen, to an appointment with his pulmonologist. In early February, while COVID-19 was establishing a beachhead in this country, my father had suffered a gastrointestinal bleed and lost a lot of blood. We had taken him to Hoag Hospital in Newport Beach, where doctors could not find the source of the bleed. His medical team should have given him a transfusion, but since they felt his anemia was not quite severe enough, they had discharged him after a week, even though he was still in a weakened state. At the time, I noticed he also had a new cough.

In the middle of March, his cough was getting worse. We were just starting the first nationwide lockdown—called "15 Days to Slow the Spread"—so this novel coronavirus was on everyone's mind. I had COVID-19 test kits at Amen Clinics and sent my niece Krystle, who was the clinic director for our Costa Mesa office, to my parents' home to have them tested.

Two days later, we discovered that both my parents tested positive. Paramedics whisked them to Hoag, where the hospital arranged for my parents to share a room. We weren't allowed to visit them, however, and wondered if we would ever see them again this side of heaven. This happened at a time when images of forklifts loading dead bodies into refrigerator trucks parked outside New York City hospitals were dominating the news coverage.

My parents were put on a regimen of hydrochloroquine, azithromycin, and zinc. My mom was part of a clinical trial where she was randomized to receive either hydroxychloroquine and azithromycin or remdesivir. My wife, Tana, and I laughed with Mom when she told us over the phone that she had to sign an agreement not to get pregnant during the treatment. Perhaps my mother's playful sense of humor was one of the reasons she recovered almost immediately. Five days later, they were both released from the hospital and became local celebrities when the *Orange County Register* put them on the front page as an elderly success story.

Yet my dad's recovery lagged. He never gained back his energy or vitality and was sleeping up to 16 hours a day. Doctors ordered chest X-rays and put him on an antibiotic, but he was clearly not himself.

I was getting ready to leave the house on May 5 when Mom called me on my cell. She was in a panic.

"He's stopped breathing!" she cried out.

"Stay on the line. I'll call 911!" I replied.

After describing the situation to the local emergency services and giving them my parents' address, I jumped into my car and raced to their home, listening to Mom on speakerphone.

"Louie, get up," I heard her say to my father. "Louie, wake up."

I've never driven the four miles between our homes any faster. I arrived just after the paramedics pulled into my parents' driveway. When I rushed into the family room, I saw Dad lying on his back with an intubation tube down his throat.

"He has no heart rate," an EMT told me. "Do you want us to revive him?"

I didn't hesitate. "Of course," I said.

Meanwhile, Mom was obsessing. "He was fine and having a great day. I went to get dressed, and when I came back, he wasn't breathing."

"How long?" I asked my mother.

My mother shook her head. She didn't know. While paramedics performed CPR, a Newport Beach Police Department (NBPD) officer entered the house. I recognized him— Officer David Darling, an NBPD veteran. I'd met him and many of the fine police officers during my monthly visits to the NBPD headquarters, where I volunteered my time giving two-hour seminars on brain health. I wanted our police force to have healthy brains, as they definitely had a chronically stressful occupation. My friend Jon Lewis, the NBPD Chief, had the same vision as I did.

Officer Darling pulled my mother and me to the side. In a voice filled with compassion, he said, "I'm sorry to tell you this, but when someone dies at home, we have to do an investigation."

Mom's eyes got big. "Do you think I killed him? That I was cheating on him?" My mother knew she was being ridiculous; her sly smile gave her away. We all knew that a police investigation of a 90-year-old man who stopped breathing inside his home during a worldwide pandemic didn't make sense, but those were the rules.

"Mrs. Amen, we just have to follow procedure." That was the start of a terrible, horrible, no-good, very bad day, which went by in a blur. Even though we were under California's severe lockdown orders, within 90 minutes three dozen people arrived at Mom's house to comfort her and our family, including nearly all my siblings and their spouses and partners.

That evening, after a long, emotional day of

dealing with the mortuary and then watching my father's body being taken away on a gurney, I showered and got ready for bed.

For the last three or four years, I had a ritual of putting myself to sleep by saying a prayer and then asking myself, "What went well today?" This was a bookend to how I start every day by saying to myself as soon as my feet hit the floor in the morning, "Today is going to be a great day." I had embraced these twin measures of positivity bias training, because I program my mind to look for what is right, more than what is wrong. I want to focus on why it will be a great day each morning and what went well when my head hits the pillow. Training my brain to search for the good things that happened during the day was kind of like making my own highlight show. It's my habit, ritual, and routine. It is what I do.

When it was time to fall asleep that night, I said a prayer, and then my mind went to *What went well today?* Then all of sudden, my mind objected. My mind said, *Seriously, you are going to do that tonight, on the worst day of your life in 38 years? The worst day since you lost your grandfather in 1982? If you loved your father, isn't that disrespectful?*

Yet, because it was my habit, I thought about the interaction between Officer Darling and my mother. A smile creased my lips because even in tragedy, my mother hadn't lost her sense of humor. Then I thought about the dozens of texts I got that day from my friends and my father's friends. Both he and I were loved. And before I drifted off to sleep, I remembered Tana and I sitting alone with my father in the family room saying goodbye. I was holding his hands and remembered how soft they were just before the mortuary staff took him away. Even with the tragedy, I slept well that night because I had been training my mind for years.

A couple of days later, we decided to cremate my father. Somebody went to the mortuary to retrieve his clothes, wedding ring, and paperwork. At my parents' house, I was going through the paperwork with my mother and came across a picture randomly inserted in the stack of papers of my father laying at the mortuary with a sheet up to his shoulders. Seeing the picture of my dead father bothered me for the rest of the day. I just couldn't shake the image out of my mind.

Then I remembered a technique I teach my patients called "havening" (see sidebar). I recalled the image of my father at the mortuary, along with the upsetting feeling, and then put each of my hands on the opposite shoulders and gently stroked down to my elbows repeatedly for 30 seconds. I felt calmer, like I was washing away feeling upset.

Then I asked myself, "How do you feel?"

My response was quick: "I feel better."

I did this havening technique five more times for 30 seconds each. By the time I finished, a picture that bothered me had turned into a photo I could appreciate because it was the last picture I had of my father, who was at peace.

This experience was another reminder that where I directed my mind mattered. I could use my brain to torture myself with questions—Who was the idiot who placed that photo of my dead father in that stack of papers?—or I could turn my grief into something positive, which I did.

In a world of negativity, it's good to have positivity bias training.

What Exactly Is Havening?

In the early 2000s, Dr. Ronald Ruden, an internist with a PhD in organic chemistry, developed havening, a healing technique using therapeutic touch to change pathways in the brain linked to emotional distress. Dr. Ruden theorized that certain touching techniques could help boost serotonin production in the brain, allowing us to relax and detach from an upsetting life experience. The practice of havening involves one or more of the following touch techniques:

- Rubbing the palms of your hands together, slowly, as if you're washing your hands.
- Giving yourself a hug. This technique involves placing the palms of your hands on your opposite shoulders and rubbing them down your arms to your elbows.
- "Washing your face" by placing your fingertips up high on your forehead, just below your hairline, and then letting your hands fall down your face to your chin.

From a neuroscience perspective, havening is a form of stimulating both sides of the brain (essential for healing) while you mentally bring up a stressful thought or past trauma.

Havening got a boost during the pandemic when singer Justin Bieber released a YouTube documentary video showing him using the touch technique. While

Justin massages his temples in a hunched-over, sitting posture, his wife, Hailey, explains on-camera, "It's basically a self-soothing thing . . . when you're starting to feel really stressed out or just [want] to keep yourself calm. It's almost like, I think, when you're a kid, and your mom is rubbing your back to sleep, and it's the best feeling in the world. It's kind of like that, except you're doing it for yourself."[1]

Dr. Ruden reports that his research has shown that havening generates high amplitude neural oscillations known as delta waves, which we experience when asleep.[2] Delta waves calm regions of the brain involved in creating emotionally charged memories and trauma. One of these brain regions is the amygdala, which plays a significant role in recording the emotions of our experiences.

When it comes to traumatic experiences, the amygdala encodes the related emotions differently, becoming what neuroscientists call "potentiated." This means the trauma and emotions get hardwired into your brain and stick like superglue. Havening helps loosen the glue in your brain.

Introducing the Power of Positivity

Saying, "Today is going to be a great day" and employing havening techniques are examples of positivity bias training exercises that can help eliminate or suck the energy out of bad moments and bad memories.

Dr. Martin Seligman influenced me in this area. When he was elected president of the American Psychological Association more than 25 years ago, he gathered a dozen top psychologists and asked them to help him develop a plan to move the discipline of psychology away from treating mental illness and toward human flourishing. For many years, psychology worked within the disease model—treating those with mental problems and psychopathological issues. In their rush to do something about repairing mental health damage, it had never occurred to psychologists to develop positive interventions that made people happier. That was the impetus for Dr. Seligman to work with Dr. Mihaly Csikszentmihalyi and other top psychologists on a strategy they called "positive psychology," which shifted the focus of interventions from problems to solutions.

They determined that positive psychology had five key aspects:

1. Positive psychology helps us look at life with optimism.

2. Positive psychology allows us to appreciate the present.

3. Positive psychology lets us accept and make peace with the past.

4. Positive psychology helps us be more grateful and forgiving.

5. Positive psychology helps us look beyond the momentary pleasures and pains of life.[3]

Dr. Seligman introduced the concept of positive psychology at the annual American Psychological Association convention in 1998. His message: The field of psychology needed to expand its myopic focus on treating mental illness to include mental health. Then Dr. Seligman exuded transparency when he told this story before a room filled with his colleagues:

I was out weeding in my garden last summer with my daughter, Nicki, who had turned five, some 11 months earlier. Now, you should know that I'm a very serious gardener, and this particular afternoon, I'm very focused on what

I'm doing—which is weeding. Nicki, on
the other hand, is having fun. Weeds are
flying up in the air, and dirt is spraying
everywhere.

Now, I should mention here, that
despite all my work on optimism, I've
always been somewhat of a nimbus cloud
around my house. And despite all my
work with children, and despite having
five children of my own, ages five to 29,
I'm really not that good with kids. And
so, kneeling that afternoon in my garden,
I yelled at Nicki.

Nicki got a stern look on her face,
and she walked right over to me.
"Daddy," she said, "I want to talk with
you." And this is just what she said.
"From the time I was three until I was
five, I whined a lot. But I decided the
day I turned five, to stop whining. And
I haven't whined once since the day I
turned five."

Then Nicki looked me right in the eye,
and said "Daddy, if I could stop whining,
you can stop being such a grouch."[4]

The room erupted with laughter. Out of the mouths of babes, right?

With Dr. Seligman leading the charge, positive psychology started to change the landscape of psychology during the 2000s. In the past, scientists and psychologists have said that happiness is too subjective, too broad, and too culturally relative to explore seriously, but researchers have found that about 40 percent of a person's sense of positivity is due to their genetic makeup. The rest is all highly dependent on an individual's experiences, emotions, and thoughts.

Their studies also suggested that happiness could be achieved through various channels such as:

- social awareness (being aware of the physical senses of touch, smell, taste, hearing, and sight)
- social communication (verbal and nonverbal forms of social interaction)
- gratitude practices (expressing and showing heartfelt appreciation)
- cognitive reformations (changing the way you think)

Taken together, these factors are clustered in practical techniques called positive psychology interventions, or PPIs.[5] These scientific tools and strategies are designed to boost happiness, well-being, and emotions.

Positivity Bias Training Exercises: Nine Steps to Raise Your Happiness

Drs. Seligman and Csikszentmihalyi found that positive psychology interventions enhance one's life, regardless of one's mental state or circumstances. Now let's turn these interventions into nine actionable steps I teach my patients to help them be happier and overcome negative feelings.

1. **Start each morning by saying, "Today is going to be a great day."** I recommended this practice in the last chapter, noting that where you bring your attention determines how you feel. If you want to feel happier, start the day by directing your attention to what you are excited about, what you like, what you want, what you hope for, and what makes you happy, rather than the negative. I recommend families do this together as parents are

waking up their kids, or as they all sit down at the breakfast table in the morning. I love this exercise so much that it's at the top of my daily to-do list, just in case I miss saying it.

Now, I understand that saying, "Today is going to be a great day" may sound a bit, shall I say, Pollyannaish, especially during the pandemic when thousands were dying from COVID-19 or restaurant owners were forced to close their businesses. My heart grieves for those families personally hit with the coronavirus (mine included), yet being negative won't help anyone. We have a lot to do at Amen Clinics helping the thousands of people with mounting anxiety, depression, and suicidal thoughts.

By saying, "Today is going to be a great day," I have protected and focused my mind to see what is right, not just what is wrong, which is so easy to find. This helped me do hundreds of live chats on social media during the pandemic, encouraging our patients and followers.

Another reason I recommend this practice is because it plants seeds of optimism

Into the soil of everyday life. Happy individuals look for the good that can come out of a situation, not what can go wrong. One of my favorite sayings is: "A pessimist sees the difficulty in every opportunity; an optimist sees the opportunity in every difficulty."

Optimists and pessimists approach problems differently. Optimists generally proceed with a positive outlook, while pessimists expect the sky to fall. Optimists know that things don't always go their way, so when life knocks them down, they get back up and try again. A sense of optimism lifts the immune system, helps prevent chronic disease, and gives you a better chance of coping with bad news, such as when my father passed away.

2. **Record your micro-moments of happiness for later viewing.** Happiness doesn't have to be something "big" or "off the chart." Happiness stemming from small moments can actually be more valuable than significant milestones like your birthday, a graduation ceremony, or a party.

By getting into the habit of looking for

and finding the teeny-tiny, itty-bitty, micro-moments of happiness throughout your day, you train your brain to have a positivity bias. Keep a written journal or use the notes section of your phone to record these moments throughout your day. Then, refer to them at the end of your day to make sure you don't miss out on the little things that help you feel happy. When you really pay attention to these micro-moments, they can have a big impact on your chemicals of happiness and overall positivity. "Seek and you will find" (Matthew 7:7, NIV).

> *Happiness stemming from small moments can actually be more valuable than significant milestones.*

3. **Express gratitude and appreciation as often as possible.** Behavioral scientist Steve Maraboli, the author of *Unapologetically You*, published a gratitude journal in 2020 called *If You Want to Find Happiness Find Gratitude.*[6] And why not? As I discussed in the last chapter, we feel more positive when we express gratitude.

Focusing on gratitude boosts your happiness, health, appearance, and relationships. Appreciation brings gratitude to a new level because it builds bridges between people. Write down three things you are grateful for each day and try to find one person to appreciate. This simple exercise can make a significant difference in your level of happiness in just a few short weeks.

Dr. Seligman came up with a practice to enhance people's happiness called "The Gratitude Visit." This is how he described it:

> Close your eyes. Call up the face of someone still alive who years ago did something or said something that changed your life for the better. Someone who you never properly thanked; someone you could meet face-to-face next week. Got a face?
>
> Gratitude can make your life happier and more satisfying. When we feel gratitude, we benefit from the pleasant memory of a positive event in our life. Also, when we express our

gratitude to others, we strengthen our relationship with them. But sometimes our thank-you is said so casually or quickly that it is nearly meaningless. In this exercise . . . you will have the opportunity to experience what it is like to express your gratitude in a thoughtful, purposeful manner.

Your task is to write a letter of gratitude to this individual and deliver it in person. The letter should be concrete and about 300 words: be specific about what she did for you and how it affected your life. Let her know what you are doing now, and mention how you often remember what she did. Make it sing! Once you have written the testimonial, call the person and tell her you'd like to visit her, but be vague about the purpose of the meeting; this exercise is much more fun when it is a surprise. When you meet her, take your time reading your letter.[7]

Dr. Seligman says that if you're able to read this testimonial in person, be prepared: You'll set off some waterworks. Everyone weeps when a gratitude letter is read. When Dr. Seligman tested those who participated in a gratitude letter one week, one month, and three months later, they were both happier and less depressed.

4. **Show empathy and kindness to others.** When we seek to understand another person's perspective, we better understand his or her feelings as well. Self-love meditations and mindfulness practices are two exercises that promote empathy and positive feelings toward ourselves and others. Effective communication and more informed perceptions help us create meaningful connections.

   A lot of people have or are going through tough times these days. Is there someone you could call or video chat with to ask how he or she is doing? Is there someone you know who needs someone to talk to?

   Research shows that kindness leads to happiness. We've all heard the term "random acts of kindness," those selfless actions performed by people to help or encourage a stranger for no other reason than to put a smile on someone's face. There are dozens of ways to show kindness, but here are a few ideas:

- Smile when you see someone walking toward you.
- Hold the door open for someone and be less in a hurry.
- Be a good listener.
- Ask the person who is serving you how his or her day is going and listen.
- Send flowers to a friend.
- Send a funny cartoon or joke to a friend.
- Spend time playing with your pet.

Gestures of altruism have been shown to increase both the giver's and receiver's well-being. However, research led by Timothy D. Windsor, PhD, at the Centre for Mental Health Research at Australian National

University, showed that individuals who spent *too little* or *too much* time volunteering reported similarly low levels of well-being. Those who spent a moderate amount of time volunteering reported the highest levels of life satisfaction.[8]

Along those lines, I use an acronym for those I hire at Amen Clinics and BrainMD (a nutraceutical company), and it comes from one of my favorite former Los Angeles Lakers players, Kentavious Caldwell-Pope, who plays with such infectious energy and enthusiasm. On the way home from attending a Lakers game where Kentavious played well and seemed to be having so much fun, I thought of wanting team members who were just like him—KCP: Kind, Competent, and Passionate. That has truly helped the culture of our teams at Amen Clinics. We focus on kindness, competence, and being passionate about brain health.

5. **Focus on your strengths and accomplishments.** An essential virtue of positive psychological interventions is focusing on what's

right rather than what's wrong. Likewise, focusing on your strengths rather than your weaknesses is essential. Dr. Seligman participated in a 2005 study demonstrating that strength-based interventions boosted happiness and reduced depressive symptoms after just a month. However, it's critical that a person actually *use* the identified strengths. Simply talking about them doesn't yield the same benefits.[9]

What are five things you're good at? If you aren't sure, what are five things your friends say you do well?

When you have written something down, think of ways to use those attributes in your everyday life. For instance, you may have grown up in a bilingual home and have a proficiency in another language. Could you be putting that skill to better use in your career? The same goes for computer expertise, an ability to cook, or an ability to lead teams. Your personal skills can become your signature strengths.

A key to focusing on your strengths is having the right expectations and aspirations.

It's interesting how, from a young age, we hear the myth that we can become anything we want to be, even the president of the United States. We move into the adult years with lofty expectations and hopes for a bright future, but if we learned anything from recent history, it's that we can't expect *anything* these days.

You will increase your happiness if you scrap or reduce any unrealistic expectations. Chances are you're not going to have the perfect career, the perfect spouse, or the perfect kids. In fact, seeking perfection is a recipe for unhappiness because you will always be disappointed. Set expectations that make sense to the current situation you find yourself in. And match those expectations with what you've learned about yourself through a strengths-based assessment.

Likewise, focus on your accomplishments. What have you achieved? When I asked one of my patients this question, he answered with "I can't keep a relationship." He had been married 11 times. Using positivity bias training, we reframed the situation

to show him that he was very good at starting relationships and getting women to fall
in love with him. We were going to work on
how the relationships could last. We noticed
what was right and then focused on what
could be improved.

What have you accomplished? Write it
down. Look at it. I keep a file on my phone
of cool events I've participated in or hosted,
and I look at it whenever I feel down.

6. **Train yourself to live in the present moment.**
    We've all heard the stock phrases like "Live in
    the here and now" or "Make the most of each
    day," but research shows that happy people
    live more fully in the moment than those who
    are unhappy. A pair of Harvard researchers
    put this concept to the test when they cre-
    ated an app to analyze people's minute-by-
    minute thoughts, feelings, and actions.[10]
    What they discovered is that unhappy people
    tend to think about what is *not* happening as
    much as they think about what *is* happening
    in the current moment—and this typically
    makes them unhappy. Conversely, happy

people who focus on the present are not pre
occupied with past hurts, stressed by regret,
or wrapped up in what might happen in the
future. Instead, their attention is focused on
the present moment, meaning they are aware
and mindful of what is happening right now.

Being present-minded is critical to health
and happiness. It will ground you and ensure
you remain connected to the world around
you. This doesn't mean you empty your mind
of all thoughts, but your attention is focused
on what you're doing, who you're with, and
what you're experiencing.

I happened to read the book *The Power
of Now*, written by Eckhart Tolle, after I
had lost someone important to me and I
was grieving. The pain caused me to hunt
through past memories, which filled me with
regret, anxiety, and chest pain. My gut was
not cooperating, and I was miserable. The
most important concept I took from *The
Power of Now* was that my thoughts were
causing me to suffer as I allowed repetitive
thoughts to steal my vital energy. If I wasn't
mentally preparing myself for something

that would happen in the future, then I was getting lost in the past. But the more I lived in the present moment, the more I felt free from the emotional pain of the past and the worries about the future.

Present moment thinking is important even during hard times. While we want to get away from or escape pain, we must go *into* the pain. In my book *Your Brain Is Always Listening*, I wrote about the importance of allowing grief to wash over you and to let your tears flow in times of loss.[11] When we acknowledge and go into our pain, it starts to dissipate. By being present and mindful of where we are, we are more apt to feel happy and secure, better handle pain, reduce the impact of stress on our health, and better cope with challenging emotions.[12]

Here's one thing I've done to focus my mind on the present moment. On several consecutive occasions, each time I sat down in my car, I'd feel the steering wheel before I turned on the engine. I would grip the wheel, noting my hand position and the molded material around the rim. Spending a good 20 or 30 seconds on this before driving off was a slowing-life-down exercise that allowed me to "anchor" myself to the present moment. By observing my hands and observing my breathing, I connected my body and mind in the here and now.

Who doesn't need a reminder to grip a steering wheel or smell the roses as we rush through life? When we choose to savor the world around us—from breathing in the comforting smell of fresh laundry coming out of the dryer or slowly enjoying the intricate tastes of food—we refresh our sensory experiences.

Part of living in the present means not worrying about the future, which will kill your happiness every day of the week and twice on Sunday. Worrying may be second nature to many, but most of us are not aware of how much we dwell on fearful thoughts. Research shows that happy people worry far less often than unhappy people do.[13] This insight isn't new, however. In fact, there's a wonderful passage on this concept in the Bible:

Therefore I tell you, do not worry about your life, what you will eat or drink; or about your body, what you will wear. Is not life more than food, and the body more than clothes? Look at the birds of the air; they do not sow or reap or store away in barns, and yet your heavenly Father feeds them. Are you not much more valuable than they? Can any one of you by worrying add a single hour to your life?

MATTHEW 6:25-27, NIV

7. **Be positive by eliminating the negative.** As much as we want to think positively, our brains love to camp out in negative territories—what I call the Badlands. Early in my practice, I treated so many patients complaining about deep, dark, negative thoughts that it was like they were on automatic pilot, sharing their negative thoughts reflexively.

Most people don't know that positive and negative thoughts release different chemicals in the brain. Whenever you have a happy thought, a bright idea, or a loving feeling, your brain releases the chemicals of happiness, such as dopamine, serotonin, and endorphins that calm the body. Whenever you have a negative thought, the brain releases or decreases chemicals, leaving you angry, sad, or stressed out. The release of stress hormones, cortisol and adrenaline, and the depletion of feel-good neurotransmitters (dopamine and serotonin) changes your body's chemistry and brain's focus. This makes you unhappy.

It's hard to climb the ladder of happiness when negativity is pulling at your legs. Sure, life is filled with problems, heartbreaks, and disappointments. Bad things happen both personally and professionally. Relationships end, and friends and family members die. It's important to grieve losses, such as I did with my father, and grief can be better dealt with when you give yourself time and space to do so. Realize that it may be weeks or months before you return to roughly the same level of happiness that you had before.

What you can control is how you react to the inevitable negative things that happen to you. Challenge your thoughts to achieve a more positive outlook.

8. **Find fun and laughter in your life.** Want to inject a little positivity into your life? Laugh more. Every time you let out a chuckle, your brain releases the chemicals of happiness—dopamine, oxytocin, and endorphins—while lowering the stress hormone cortisol. A hearty laugh is like a drug, changing your brain chemistry to make you feel happier, and making it happen almost instantly.

However, laughter is in short supply these days, especially the older we become. "The collective loss of our sense of humor is a serious problem afflicting people and organizations globally," contend Jennifer Aaker and Naomi Bagdonas, authors of *Humor, Seriously*. They point to a Gallup Poll involving 1.4 million people in 166 countries showing that the frequency with which we laugh or smile each day starts to plummet around age 23.[14] This explains why adults laugh an average of 4.2 times a day, which is a fraction of the giggles, chuckles, and bursts of laughter from children, who laugh an average of 300 times a day.

So what is laughter, and how does it happen? Laughter shows emotion, such as mirth, joy, or scorn with a chuckle or explosive vocal sound.

What this definition lacks is where laughter *starts*, and that's the brain. We know that the left side of the brain is responsible for interpreting words, including jokes. The brain's right side is responsible for identifying what makes the joke, observation, or situation funny. The brain's prefrontal cortex is responsible for emotional responses, but don't forget that the basal ganglia—the area of the brain that integrates movement and emotion—becomes active when we're watching a funny movie or sitcom on TV. These areas produce the physical actions of laughing.

The best thing about laughter is how good it is for you. A Loma Linda University study on the effect of laughter showed that hilarity and mirth release endorphins—the body's painkillers—and lower blood pressure.[15] As the old proverb goes, laughter is the best medicine, and "humor is mankind's greatest blessing"—a famous saying attributed to Mark Twain.

So how can you laugh more? Well, laughter is contagious, so if you and your friends are able to take in a comedy at the movies, visit a local comedy club, or watch a live production of a farce-type play, do it. If everyone is laughing together, a bond is created that makes you more likely to express your true feelings, which also has a positive effect on your life.

In *Humor, Seriously*, Aaker and Bagdonas write that using humor to make other people laugh can be just as beneficial, helping us appear more intelligent, deepening bonds, enhancing creativity, and strengthening resilience. So how can you make others laugh if you weren't born with a natural funny bone? With practice, even you can find your wittiness by using two common elements of humor:

- A foundation in the truth
- The unexpected

I often use these two principles of humor in my clinical practice as well as in my books and public television shows. It allows me to deliver complex information in a way that helps people understand it and remember it more easily. For example, here is something I said in my public television show *Change Your Brain, Heal Your Mind.*

I was telling the audience that it was my fourteenth public television show about the brain and that everywhere I go across the country people tell me how my programs have changed their lives. So I gave them the following few examples:

I was walking recently when I saw a couple running toward me. The wife recognized me and said, "Hey, you're the brain doctor. We are out here running because of you. My husband wouldn't listen to *me*, but he listens to *you!*"

I also met a flight attendant who told me that she lost 30 pounds and stopped feeling depressed since watching my shows because she completely changed her diet and was getting her husband and her children to walk with her.

And I met a Stanford professor who told me he completely stopped drinking because of my programs and now wakes up feeling 100 percent every day.

Then I threw in a zinger:

But my favorite story is of the 87-year-old woman who told me that she started dating again after she watched my shows because she realized that being alone was not good for her brain. With a smile she told me that she had recently met a wonderful 80-year-old man online and they were having the time of their lives. I wondered if that qualified her as being a grandmother cougar.

As soon as I said "grandmother cougar," the audience burst out into laughter. What

I said was all rooted in truth, but I threw in something unexpected that made the audience's brains do a double take. And by making them laugh, my own brain released a cocktail of feel-good neurochemicals that made me feel happy at the same time.

9. **End your day by asking yourself,** *What went well today?* I've already described how I've been using this example of positivity bias training in my own life, especially the day I lost my father. You don't have to wait until your head hits the pillow to ask yourself what went well. This is an excellent exercise that any family can do around the dinner table and something we do in the Amen home.

A couple of years ago, two of my nieces came to live with us because their parents were caught up in addictions, and Tana and I wanted to provide them with a healthier home environment. At breakfast we ask them, "So why is today going to be a great day?" And at dinner we talk about what went well. That's how I recommend families do it. Find a consistent time every day to point the day in a positive direction and wrap up the day by reviewing what went well.

I can always find something that went well each day, and so can you, even during tough times. Looking for the good things that happened during your waking hours will train your brain to search for ESPN-like "Plays of the Day." It doesn't matter if those plays are spectacular, good, average, or routine—they are yours. Thinking about the good things that happened to you sets up your dreams to be more positive, which will help you sleep better, enhance your mood, boost your energy levels, and put a smile on your face. When you fall asleep happier, you wake up happier, ready to embrace the day with a positive bias.

Life Is a Picnic

Just like the infestation that attacked my kitchen all those years ago, ANTs will assault you every day. Some days they'll be whispering inside your head. Other days they'll be screaming incessantly. You'll know they are running wild if they are impairing how you think, feel, or act. But If you practice the techniques we've discussed in this book, you can identify and squash those ANTs before they get out of control!

Better yet, if you not only squash those ANTs, but replace them with positive, life-giving thoughts, you'll feel more confident and resilient and be fully prepared to face whatever life throws your way, whether it's the end of a relationship, the loss of a job, or an unexpected health crisis.

You'll no longer give in to negative thinking or let bad habits derail your health and relationships, even in times of trauma, extreme stress, or grief. You'll be able to recognize what's true, build your self-confidence, discipline your mind, and feel happier, calmer, and in more control of your own destiny.

Once you master these techniques, share them with others! That way you are also creating your own support group, making it more likely you will keep these new habits for the rest of your life!

Life really can be a picnic. You just need to get rid of those pesky ANTs!

HOW CHALLENGING 100 OF YOUR WORST THOUGHTS CAN CHANGE YOUR LIFE

ONE OF THE FIRST EXERCISES I give patients is to have them write down 100 of their worst ANTs. Then we subject each of them to the elimination process. If you do this with diligence and thoughtfulness, I promise you will stop the ANTs, end self-defeating thoughts, and be more in control of your happiness and destiny. The brain learns by repetition.

Undisciplined or negative thinking is like a bad habit. The more you engage in it, the more easily the ANTs will attack and take over your mind. These bad thinking habits form through a process called long-term potentiation. When neurons fire together, they wire together, and the negative thoughts become an ingrained part of your life. That is why you need to do this exercise 100 times to teach your brain a new, more rational way of thinking.

You do not have to believe every thought you have. If you want emotional freedom, it is critical to develop the skill of guiding and directing your thoughts. This is the first step in developing strong mental discipline. Whenever you feel sad, mad, nervous, or out of control, write down your ANTs, identify which type they are (there may be more than one type), and then ask yourself the following five simple questions (briefly referred to in chapter 2) that I learned from Byron Katie. They are life-changing. There are no right or wrong answers; they are just questions to open your mind to alternative possibilities. Meditate on each answer to see how it makes you feel. Ask yourself if your stressful thoughts make your life better or worse.

ANT:

ANT Type(s):

Five Questions

1. **Is it true?** Sometimes this first question will stop the ANT because you already know it's not true. Sometimes your answer will be "I don't know." If you don't know, then do not act like the negative thought is true. Sometimes you may think or feel that the negative thought is true, but that is why the second question is so important.

2. **Is it absolutely true with 100 percent certainty?**

3. How do I feel when I believe this thought?

4. How would I feel if I couldn't have this thought?

5. Turn the thought around to its exact opposite, and then ask yourself: "Any evidence that that's true?" Then use this turnaround statement as a meditation.

During the pandemic, one of my patients called in a panic because she lost her job, and she told me, "I'll never be able to work again." I guided her through the five questions to work on that thought:

ANT: *I'll never be able to work again.*

ANT Type(s): Fortune-Telling

1. **Is it true?** Yes

2. **Is it absolutely true with 100 percent certainty?** No, I already have part-time work lined up.

3. **How do I feel when I believe this thought?** Trapped, victimized, helpless

4. **How would I feel if I couldn't have this thought?** Massively relieved, happy, joyful, free, like my usual self

5. **Turn the thought around to its exact opposite:** I can get work again. **Any evidence that that's true?** I have valuable skills that will help me get a job.

Thought to meditate on: *I have valuable skills that will help me get a job.*

If you do this exercise with your most toxic thoughts, it will change your life because your brain will begin to stop listening to the negativity running through your head and start listening to the truth. Remember, this is not about positive thinking. It is about accurate thinking. To make this technique clear, here are several more examples:

FROM A MAN SUFFERING WITH SEVERE DEPRESSION

ANT: *I'm going to end up like my father who abandoned us.*

ANT Type(s): Fortune-Telling

1. **Is it true?** No

2. **Is it absolutely true with 100 percent certainty?** No, I will always be here for my children and wife.

3. **How do I feel when I believe this thought?**
Like I lost at life; I feel like a failure, scum,
sad, anxious, angry

4. **How would I feel if I couldn't have this
thought?** Relieved, free, safe

5. **Turn the thought around to its exact opposite:**
I am not going to end up like my father. **Any
evidence that that's true?** Yes, I am with my
family, employed, and not addicted to drugs.

Thought to meditate on: *I am not going to end
up like my father.*

**FROM A WOMAN WHO HAD TO TESTIFY
AGAINST A MAN WHO MURDERED HER
SON IN A BAR FIGHT**

ANT: *I'm evil because I want him to suffer.*

ANT Type(s): Labeling

1. **Is it true?** No

2. **Is it absolutely true with 100 percent certainty?** No

3. **How do I feel when I believe this thought?** Horrible, like I am a bad person. Who am I to judge others?

4. **How would I feel if I couldn't have this thought?** Still grieving my son but without self-recrimination

5. **Turn the thought around to its exact opposite:** I am not evil; I am loving. I am just going to tell the truth and allow the justice system to work. **Any evidence that that's true?** Yes, I do many helpful and loving things for other people.

Thought to meditate on: *I am loving.*

FROM A POLICE OFFICER WHO WAS STRESSED AT WORK

ANT: *I'm not making a difference.*

ANT Type(s): All-or-Nothing

1. **Is it true?** Yes

2. **Is it absolutely true with 100 percent certainty?** No

3. **How do I feel when I believe this thought?**
Useless, weak, withering, sad

4. **How would I feel if I couldn't have this thought?** Optimistic, purposeful, content, motivated, happier

5. **Turn the thought around to its exact opposite:** I am making a difference. **Any evidence that that's true?** Yes, every day I have good interactions that help others.

Thought to meditate on: *I am making a difference.*

FROM A STATE DEPARTMENT EMPLOYEE WHO WAS STRUGGLING WITH COWORKERS

ANT: *The more you do, the more you get screwed.*

ANT Type(s): Just-the-Bad

1. **Is it true?** Yes

2. **Is it absolutely true with 100 percent certainty?** No

3. **How do I feel when I believe this thought?** Angry, useless, unmotivated

4. **How would I feel if I couldn't have this thought?** Purposeful, happy, more present and in the moment

5. **Turn the thought around to its exact opposite:** The more I do, the less I get screwed. **Any evidence that that's true?** Yes, the more I do, the more I help and live my purpose.

Thought to meditate on: *The more I do, the more I help and live my purpose.*

FROM A WIDOWED MOTHER OF FOUR CHILDREN WHO WAS CHRONICALLY STRESSED AND UNHAPPY BUT NOT ASKING FOR HELP FROM HER FAMILY.

ANT: *I should be the strong one.*

ANT Type(s): Guilt-Beating

1. **Is it true?** Yes

2. **Is it absolutely true with 100 percent certainty?** No. At this pace, I am unable to do it all myself.

3. **How do I feel when I believe this thought?** Defeated, depressed, overwhelmed, like running away

4. **How would I feel if I couldn't have this thought?** Like a good mother because I would ask for help and have it when I needed it.

5. **Turn the thought around to its exact opposite:** I don't have to be the only strong one. I can ask for help. **Any evidence that's true?** Yes, my family has offered, and I can accept their help with gratitude.

Thought to meditate on: *I can ask for help.*

See how easy it is? Now try a few of your own!

ANT: _____

ANT Type(s): _____

1. Is it true? _____

2. Is it absolutely true with 100 percent certainty? _____

3. How do I feel when I believe this thought?

   _____

   _____

   _____

4. How would I feel if I couldn't have this thought? _____

   _____

   _____

5. Turn the thought around to its exact opposite: _____

   _____

   _____

   _____

   _____

   _____

Thought to meditate on: _____

_____

_____

_____

_____

_____

_____

_____

_____

ANT: _____

ANT Type(s): _____

1. Is it true? _____

2. Is it absolutely true with 100 percent certainty? _____

3. How do I feel when I believe this thought?

   _____

   _____

   _____

4. How would I feel if I couldn't have this thought? _____

   _____

   _____

5. Turn the thought around to its exact opposite: _____

   _____

   _____

   _____

   _____

Thought to meditate on: _____

_____

_____

_____

_____

_____

_____

_____

ANT: _____

ANT Type(s): _____

1. Is it true? _____

2. Is it absolutely true with 100 percent certainty? _____

3. How do I feel when I believe this thought?
   _____
   _____

4. How would I feel if I couldn't have this thought? _____
   _____
   _____

5. Turn the thought around to its exact opposite: _____
   _____
   _____
   _____
   _____
   _____
   _____

Thought to meditate on: _____

_____

_____

_____

_____

_____

_____

_____

BIBLE VERSES TO HELP CONQUER NEGATIVE THOUGHTS

IT'S VIRTUALLY IMPOSSIBLE TO be 100 percent happy all the time. But when negative thoughts do come your way, one of the easiest and most effective ways to combat them is by spending time praying and quietly meditating on God's Word. Here are 28 positive, life-giving passages from Scripture to help you refocus your mind, refresh your soul, and renew your strength.

Finally, brothers and sisters, whatever is true, whatever is noble, whatever is right, whatever is pure, whatever is lovely, whatever is admirable—if anything is excellent or praiseworthy—think about such things.

PHILIPPIANS 4:8, NIV

Let all bitterness and wrath and anger and clamor and slander be put away from you, along with all malice. Be kind to one another, tenderhearted, forgiving one another, as God in Christ forgave you.

EPHESIANS 4:31-32, ESV

Do not be conformed to this world, but be transformed by the renewal of your mind, that by testing you may discern what is the will of God, what is good and acceptable and perfect.

ROMANS 12:2, ESV

Do not repay evil for evil or reviling for reviling, but on the contrary, bless, for to this you were called, that you may obtain a blessing.

I PETER 3:9, ESV

Don't worry about anything; instead, pray about everything. Tell God what you need, and thank him for all he has done. Then you will experience God's peace, which exceeds anything we can understand. His peace will guard your hearts and minds as you live in Christ Jesus.

PHILIPPIANS 4:6-7

Don't worry about tomorrow, for tomorrow will bring its own worries. Today's trouble is enough for today.

MATTHEW 6:34

Say to those with fearful hearts,
    "Be strong, and do not fear,
for your God is coming to destroy
        your enemies.
    He is coming to save you."

ISAIAH 35:4

Worry weighs a person down;
    an encouraging word cheers a person up.

PROVERBS 12:25

Humble yourselves under the mighty power of God, and at the right time he will lift you up in honor. Give all your worries and cares to God, for he cares about you.

1 PETER 5:6-7

Take my yoke upon you. Let me teach you, because I am humble and gentle at heart, and you will find rest for your souls.

MATTHEW 11:29

Can all your worries add a single moment to your life?

MATTHEW 6:27

I am leaving you with a gift—peace of mind and heart. And the peace I give is a gift the world cannot give. So don't be troubled or afraid.

JOHN 14:27

Don't be afraid, little flock. For it gives your Father great happiness to give you the Kingdom.

LUKE 12:32

The LORD is my helper,
>> so I will have no fear.
>> What can mere people
>>> do to me?

HEBREWS 13:6

There is nothing better than to be happy
and enjoy ourselves as long as we can.
And people should eat and drink and
enjoy the fruits of their labor, for these
are gifts from God.

ECCLESIASTES 3:12-13

For I know the plans I have for you,
declares the LORD, plans for welfare and
not for evil, to give you a future and
a hope.

JEREMIAH 29:11, ESV

Give your burdens to the LORD,
>> and he will take care of you.
>> He will not permit the godly to slip
>>> and fall.

PSALM 55:22

If you remain in me and my words remain in you, you may ask for anything you want, and it will be granted!

JOHN 15:7

Have faith in God. Truly, I say to you, whoever says to this mountain, "Be taken up and thrown into the sea," and does not doubt in his heart, but believes that what he says will come to pass, it will be done for him. Therefore I tell you, whatever you ask in prayer, believe that you have received it, and it will be yours. And whenever you stand praying, forgive, if you have anything against anyone, so that your Father also who is in heaven may forgive you your trespasses.

MARK 11:22-25, ESV

The LORD hears his people when
    they call to him for help.
  He rescues them from all their
    troubles.

PSALM 34:17

I am leaving you with a gift—peace of
mind and heart. And the peace I give is
a gift the world cannot give. So don't be
troubled or afraid.

JOHN 14:27

I know the LORD is always with me.
    I will not be shaken, for he is right
        beside me.

PSALM 16:8

This is the day that the LORD has made;
let us rejoice and be glad in it.

PSALM 118:24, ESV

In my distress I prayed to the LORD,
    and the LORD answered me and set me free.
The LORD is for me, so I will have no fear.
What can mere people do to me?

PSALM 118:5-6

We know that God causes everything to work
together for the good of those who love God
and are called according to his purpose.

ROMANS 8:28

This is my command—be strong
and courageous! Do not be afraid or
discouraged. For the LORD your God is
with you wherever you go.

JOSHUA 1:9

Can all your worries add a single
moment to your life?

LUKE 12:25

God has not given us a spirit of fear
and timidity, but of power, love, and
self-discipline.

2 TIMOTHY 1:7

ABOUT DANIEL G. AMEN, MD

DANIEL G. AMEN, MD, believes that brain health is central to all health and success. When your brain works right, he says, you work right, and when your brain is troubled, you are much more likely to have trouble in your life. His work is dedicated to helping people have better brains and better lives.

Sharecare named him the web's #1 most influential expert and advocate on mental health, and the *Washington Post* called him the most popular psychiatrist in America. His online videos have been viewed more than 150 million times.

Dr. Amen is a physician, board-certified child and adult psychiatrist, award-winning researcher, and 12-time *New York Times* bestselling author. He is the founder and CEO of Amen Clinics in Costa Mesa, Walnut Creek, and Encino, California; Bellevue, Washington; Washington, DC; Atlanta, GA; Chicago, IL; Dallas, TX; New York, NY; Scottsdale, AZ; and Hollywood, FL.

Amen Clinics has the world's largest database of functional brain scans relating to behavior, with more than 200,000 SPECT scans and more than 10,000 QEEGs on patients from over 155 countries.

Dr. Amen is the lead researcher on the world's largest brain imaging and rehabilitation study on professional football players. His research has not only demonstrated high levels of brain damage in players, but also the possibility of significant recovery for many with the principles that underlie his work.

Together with Pastor Rick Warren and Dr. Mark Hyman, Dr. Amen is also one of the chief architects of The Daniel Plan, a program to get the world healthy through religious organizations, which has been done in thousands of churches, mosques, and synagogues.

Dr. Amen is the author or coauthor of more than 80 professional articles, 9 book chapters, and over 40 books, including 18 national bestsellers and 12 *New York Times* bestsellers, including the #1 *New York Times* bestsellers *The Daniel Plan* and the over-one-million-copies-sold, 40-week bestseller *Change Your Brain, Change Your Life*; as well as *The End of Mental Illness*; *Healing ADD*; *Change Your Brain, Change Your Body*; *The Brain Warrior's Way*; *Memory Rescue*; *Your Brain Is Always Listening*; *You, Happier*; and *Change Your Brain Every Day*.

Dr. Amen's published scientific articles have appeared in the prestigious journals of *Journal of Alzheimer's Disease*, Nature's *Molecular Psychiatry*, *PLOS ONE*, Nature's *Translational Psychiatry*, Nature's *Obesity*, *Journal of Neuropsychiatry and Clinical Neuroscience*, *Minerva Psichiatrica*, *Journal of Neurotrauma*, *American Journal of Psychiatry*, *Nuclear Medicine Communications*, *Neurological Research*, *Journal of the American Academy of Child and Adolescent Psychiatry*, *Primary Psychiatry*, *Military Medicine*, and *General Hospital Psychiatry*.

In January 2016, his team's research on distinguishing PTSD from TBI on over 21,000 SPECT scans was featured as one of the top 100 stories in science by *Discover* magazine. In 2017, his team published a study on over 46,000 scans, showing the difference between male and female brains; and in 2018, his team published a study on how the brain ages based on 62,454 SPECT scans.

Dr. Amen has written, produced, and hosted 17 national public television programs about brain health, which have aired more than 130,000 times across North America. As of March 2023, his latest show is *Change Your Brain Every Day*.

Together with his wife, Tana, he has hosted *The Brain Warrior's Way Podcast* since 2015, with over 1,000 episodes and 14 million downloads. It has been listed as one of the top 20 all-time podcasts in Mental Health on Apple.

Dr. Amen has appeared in movies, including *Quiet Explosions*, *After the Last Round*, and *The Crash Reel* and was a consultant for *Concussion*, starring Will Smith. He appeared in the docu series *Justin Bieber: Seasons* and has appeared regularly on *The Dr. Oz Show*, *Dr. Phil*, and *The Doctors*.

He has also spoken for the National Security Agency (NSA), the National Science Foundation (NSF), Harvard's Learning and the Brain Conference, the Department of the Interior, the National Council of Juvenile and Family Court Judges, the Supreme Courts of Ohio, Delaware, and Wyoming, the Canadian and Brazilian Societies of Nuclear Medicine, and large corporations, such as Merrill Lynch, Hitachi, Bayer Pharmaceuticals, GNC, and many others. In 2016, Dr. Amen gave one of the prestigious Talks at Google.

Dr. Amen's work has been featured in *Newsweek*, *Time*, *Huffington Post*, *ABC World News*, *20/20*, the BBC, *London Telegraph*, *Parade* magazine, the *New York Times*, the *New York Times Magazine*, the *Washington Post*, *MIT Technology*, *World Economic Forum*, the *Los Angeles Times*, *Men's Health*, *Bottom Line*, *Vogue*, *Cosmopolitan*, and many others.

In 2010, Dr. Amen founded BrainMD,

a fast-growing nutraceutical company dedicated to natural ways to support mental health and brain health.

Dr. Amen is married to Tana and is the father of four children and grandfather to Elias, Emmy, Liam, Louie, and Haven. He is also an avid table tennis player.

NOTES

INTRODUCTION

1. K. McSpadden, "You Now Have a Shorter Attention Span Than a Goldfish," *Time*, May 14, 2015, http://time.com/3858309/attention-spans-goldfish/.
2. J. Twenge, "What Might Explain the Unhappiness Epidemic?" The Conversation website, January 22, 2018, https://theconversation.com/what-might-explain-the-unhappiness-epidemic-90212.
3. Dennis Prager, "Why Be Happy?" PragerU, January 20, 2014, video, https://www.youtube.com/watch?v=_Zxnw0l499g.

CHAPTER 2: YOU ARE WHAT YOU THINK

1. Natalie L. Marchant et al., "Repetitive Negative Thinking Is Associated with Amyloid, Tau, and

151

Cognitive Decline," *Alzheimer's & Dementia* 16, no. 7 (June 7, 2020): 1054–1064, https://alz-journals.onlinelibrary.wiley.com/doi/full/10.1002/alz.12116.

2. Majid Fotuhi, "Can You Grow Your Hippocampus? Yes. Here's How, and Why It Matters," SharpBrains, November 4, 2015, https://sharpbrains.com/blog/2015/11/04/can-you-grow-your-hippocampus-yes-heres-how-and-why-it-matters/.

3. Daniel Amen, *Change Your Brain, Change Your Life*, rev. ed., (New York: Harmony Books, 2015), 44, 49–55.

4. Read more about the BRIGHT MINDS risk factors in *Memory Rescue* or *The End of Mental Illness*.

5. R. F. Baumeister et al., "Bad Is Stronger Than Good," *Review of General Psychology* 5, no. 4 (December 2001): 323–370, doi: 10.1037/1089-2680.5.4.323.

6. J. McCoy, "New Outbrain Study Says Negative Headlines Do Better Than Positive," Business 2 Community website, March 15, 2014, https://www.business2community.com/blogging/new-outbrain-study-says-negative-headlines-better-positive-0810707.

7. R. Williams, "Are We Hardwired to Be Negative or Positive?" ICF website, June 30, 2014, https://coachfederation.org/are-we-hardwired-to-be-negative-or-positive/.

8. R. Hanson, "Confronting the Negativity Bias," *Rick Hanson* (blog), accessed March 25, 2018, http://www.rickhanson.net/how-your-brain-makes-you-easily-intimidated/.

9. C. A. Lengacher et al., "Immune Responses to Guided Imagery during Breast Cancer Treatment," *Biological Research for Nursing* 9, no. 3 (January 2008): 205–14, doi: 10.1177/1099800407309374.

C. Maack and P. Nolan, "The Effects of Guided Imagery and Music Therapy on Reported Change in Normal Adults," *Journal of Music Therapy* 36, no. 1 (March 1, 1999): 39–55.

A. G. Walton, "7 Ways Meditation Can Actually Change the Brain," *Forbes*, February 9, 2015, https://www.forbes.com/sites/alicegwalton/2015/02/09/7-ways-meditation-can-actually-change-the-brain/#84adaf414658.

10. H. Selye, *The Stress of Life* (New York: McGraw Hill, 1978), 418.

11. A. Amin, "31 Benefits of Gratitude: The Ultimate Science-Backed Guide," *Happier Human* website, accessed March 25, 2018, http://happierhuman.com/benefits-of-gratitude/.

12. C. Ackerman, "28 Benefits of Gratitude & Most Significant Research Findings," *Positive Psychology Program* website, April 12, 2017, https://positivepsychologyprogram.com/benefits-gratitude-research-questions/.

13. B. H. Brummett et al., "Prediction of All-Cause Mortality by the Minnesota Multiphasic Personality Inventory Optimism-Pessimism Scale Scores: Study of a College Sample during a 40-Year Follow-Up Period," *Mayo Clinic Proceedings* 81, no. 12 (December 2006): 1541–44, doi: 10.4065/81.12.1541.

14. L. S. Redwine et al., "Pilot Randomized Study of a Gratitude Journaling Intervention on Heart

Rate Variability and Inflammatory Biomarkers in Patients with Stage B Heart Failure," *Psychosomatic Medicine* 78, no. 6 (July–August 2016): 667–76, doi: 10.1097/PSY.0000000000000316.

15. K. O'Leary and S. Dockray, "The Effects of Two Novel Gratitude and Mindfulness Interventions on Well-Being," *Journal of Alternative and Complementary Medicine* 21, no. 4 (April 2015): 243–45, doi: 10.1089/acm.2014.0119.

16. S. T. Cheng et al., "Improving Mental Health in Health Care Practitioners: Randomized Controlled Trial of a Gratitude Intervention," *Journal of Consulting and Clinical Psychology* 83, no. 1 (February 2015): 177–86, doi: 10.1037 /a0037895.

17. E. Ramírez et al., "A Program of Positive Intervention in the Elderly: Memories, Gratitude and Forgiveness," *Aging and Mental Health* 18, no. 4 (May 2014): 463-70, doi: 10.1080/13607863 .2013.856858.

18. S. M. Toepfer et al., "Letters of Gratitude: Further Evidence for Author Benefits," *Journal of Happiness Studies* 13, no. 1 (March 2012): 187–201.

19. T. K. Inagaki et al., "The Neurobiology of Giving Versus Receiving Support: The Role of Stress-Related and Social Reward-Related Neural Activity," *Psychosomatic Medicine* 78, no. 4 (May 2016): 443–53, doi: 10.1097/PSY.0000000000000302.

20. J. J. Froh et al., "Counting Blessings in Early Adolescents: An Experimental Study of Gratitude and Subjective Well-Being," *Journal of School Psychology* 46, no. 2 (April 2008): 213–33, doi: 10.1016/j.jsp.2007.03.005.

21. M. E. Seligman et al., "Positive Psychology Progress: Empirical Validation of Interventions," *American Psychologist* 60, no. 5 (July–August 2005): 410–21, doi: 10.1037/0003-066X.60.5.410.

22. K. Rippstein-Leuenberger et al., "A Qualitative Analysis of the Three Good Things Intervention in Healthcare Workers," *BMJ Open* 7, no. 5 (June 13, 2017): e015826, doi: 10.1136/bmjopen-2017-015826.

23. M. Seligman, *Flourish: A Visionary New Understanding of Happiness and Well-Being* (New York: Free Press, 2011).

24. S. Wong, "Always Look on the Bright Side of Life," *Guardian*, August 11, 2009, https://www.theguardian.com/science/blog/2009/aug/11/optimism-health-heart-disease.

    H. A. Tindle et al., "Optimism, Cynical Hostility, and Incident Coronary Heart Disease and Mortality in the Women's Health Initiative," *Circulation* 120, no. 8 (August 25, 2009): 656–62, doi: 10.1161/CIRCULATIONAHA.108.827642.

    R. Hernandez et al., "Optimism and Cardiovascular Health: Multi-Ethnic Study of Atherosclerosis (MESA)," *Health Behavior and Policy Review* 2, no. 1 (January 2015): 62–73, doi: 10.14485/HBPR.2.1.6.

25. Mayo Clinic, "Mayo Clinic Study Finds Optimists Report a Higher Quality of Life than Pessimists," *ScienceDaily*, August 13, 2002, https://www.sciencedaily.com/releases/2002/08/020813071621.htm.

    C. Conversano et al., "Optimism and Its Impact on Mental and Physical Well-Being," *Clinical Practice and Epidemiology in Mental Health* 6 (2010): 25–29, doi: 10.2174/1745017901006010025.

    Harvard Men's Health Watch, "Optimism and

Your Health," *Harvard Health Publishing*, May 1, 2008, https://www.health.harvard.edu/heart-health/optimism-and-your-health.

26. E. S. Kim et al., "Dispositional Optimism Protects Older Adults from Stroke: 'The Health and Retirement Study," *Stroke* 42, no. 10 (October 2011): 2855–59, doi: 10.1161/STROKEAHA.111.613448.

27. Association for Psychological Science, "Optimism Boosts the Immune System," *ScienceDaily,* March 24, 2010, www.sciencedaily.com/releases/2010/03/100323121757.htm.

28. B. R. Goodin and H. W. Bulls, "Optimism and the Experience of Pain: Benefits of Seeing the Glass as Half Full," *Current Pain and Headache Reports* 17, no. 5 (May 2013): 329, doi: 10.1007/s11916-013-0329-8.

29. International Association for the Study of Lung Cancer, "Lung Cancer Patients with Optimistic Attitudes Have Longer Survival, Study Finds," *ScienceDaily*, March 8, 2010, www.sciencedaily.com/releases/2010/03/100303131656.htm.

30. University of California, Riverside, "Keys to Long Life? Not What You Might Expect," *ScienceDaily*, March 12, 2011, https://www.sciencedaily.com/releases/2011/03/110311153541.htm.

31. V. Venkatraman et al., "Sleep Deprivation Biases the Neural Mechanisms Underlying Economic Preferences," *Journal of Neuroscience* 31, no. 10 (March 9, 2011): 3712–18, doi: 10.1523/JNEUROSCI.4407-10.2011.

32. A. J. Dillard et al., "The Dark Side of Optimism: Unrealistic Optimism about Problems with

Alcohol Predicts Subsequent Negative Event Experiences," *Personality and Social Psychology Bulletin* 35, no. 11 (November 2009): 1540–50, doi: 10.1177/0146167209343124.

33. R. Ligneul et al., "Shifted Risk Preferences in Pathological Gambling," *Psychological Medicine* 43, no. 5 (May 2013): 1059–68, doi: 10.1017/S0033291712001900.

34. C. M. Karns et al., "The Cultivation of Pure Altruism via Gratitude: A Functional MRI Study of Change with Gratitude Practice," *Frontiers in Human Neuroscience* 11 (December 2017): article 599, doi: 10.3389/fnhum.2017.00599.

35. Michael Wines, "In Memoir, Barbara Bush Recalls Private Trials of a Political Life," *New York Times*, September 8, 1994, http://www.nytimes.com/1994/09/08/us/in-memoir-barbara-bush-recalls-private-trials-of-a-political-life.html.
    "Barbara Bush Says She Fought Depression in '76," *Washington Post*, May 20, 1990, https://www.washingtonpost.com/archive/politics/1990/05/20/barbara-bush-says-she-fought-depression-in-76/0ac40655-923e-448d-bfcc-aa3ea5cb88c0/?utm_term=.1bb20fdb6707.

36. K. E. Buchanan and A. Bardi, "Acts of Kindness and Acts of Novelty Affect Life Satisfaction," *Journal of Social Psychology* 150, no. 3 (May–June 2010): 235–37, doi: 10.1080/00224540903365554.

37. L. B. Aknin et al, "Happiness Runs in a Circular Motion: Evidence for a Positive Feedback Loop between Prosocial Spending and Happiness," *Journal of Happiness Studies* 13, no. 2 (April 2012): 347–55, doi: 10.1007/s10902-011-9267-5.

38. S. Q. Park et al., "A Neural Link between Generosity and Happiness," *Nature Communications* 8 (2017): 159674, doi: 10.1038/ncomms15964.

   S. G. Post, "Altruism, Happiness, and Health: It's Good to Be Good," *International Journal of Behavioral Medicine* 12, no. 2 (2005): 66–77, doi: 10.1207/s15327558ijbm1202_4.

   L. B. Aknin et al., "Giving Leads to Happiness in Young Children," *PLoS One* 7, no. 6 (2012): e39211, doi: 10.1371/journal.pone.0039211.

CHAPTER 3: THE POWER OF POSITIVITY

1. Justin Bieber: Seasons (YouTube Originals, 2020), season 1, episode 9, "Album on the Way," February 17, 2020, video, https://www.youtube.com/watch?v=pWcI-BeQqls&t=361s.

   Kerry Breen, "What Is Havening? Experts Weigh In on Justin Bieber's Stress-Relieving Technique," TODAY.com, March 3, 2020, https://www.today.com/health/what-havening-experts-weigh-justin-bieber-s-stress-relieving-technique-t174747.

2. Havening Techniques, "Havening Touch," https://www.havening.org/about-havening/havening-touch.

3. Madhuleena Roy Chowdhury, "19 Best Positive Psychology Interventions + How to Apply Them," PositivePsychology.com, updated May 4, 2021, https://positivepsychology.com/positive-psychology-interventions/.

4. Rob Hirtz, "Martin Seligman's Journey from Learned Helplessness to Learned Happiness," *Pennsylvania Gazette*, January 4, 1999, https://www.upenn.edu/gazette/0199/hirtz.html.

5. Chowdhury, "19 Best Positive Psychology Interventions."

6. Steve Maraboli, *If You Want to Find Happiness Find Gratitude* (self-pub., 2020).

7. Martin E.P. Seligman, *Flourish* (New York: Free Press, 2011), chapter 2.

8. Timothy D. Windsor, Kaarin J. Anstey, and Bryan Rodgers, "Volunteering and Psychological Well-Being among Young-Old Adults: How Much Is Too Much?" *Gerontologist* 48, no. 1 (February 2008): 59–70, https://pubmed.ncbi.nlm.nih.gov/18381833/.

9. Bryant M. Stone and Acacia C. Parks, "Cultivating Subjective Well-Being through Positive Psychological Interventions," in *Handbook of Well-Being*, ed. Ed Diener, Shigehiro Oishi, and Louis Tay (Salt Lake City: DEF Publishers, 2018), https://www.nobascholar.com/chapters/59/download.pdf.

10. Matthew A. Killingsworth and Daniel T. Gilbert, "A Wandering Mind Is an Unhappy Mind," *Science* 330, no. 6006 (November 12, 2010): 932, https://pubmed.ncbi.nlm.nih.gov/21071660/.

11. Daniel G. Amen, *Your Brain Is Always Listening* (Carol Stream, IL: Tyndale, 2021), 63–64.

12. Courtney E. Ackerman, "How to Live in the Moment: 35+ Tools to Be More Present," PositivePsychology.com, updated January 30, 2021, https://positivepsychology.com/present-moment/.

13. Ackerman, "How to Live in the Present Moment."

14. Jennifer Aaker and Naomi Bagdonas, *Humor, Seriously: Why Humor Is a Secret Weapon in Business and Life* (New York: Currency, 2021), 22.

15. Janelle Ringer, "Laughter: A Fool-Proof Prescription," Loma Linda University Health, April 1, 2019, https://news.llu.edu/research /laughter-fool-proof-prescription.

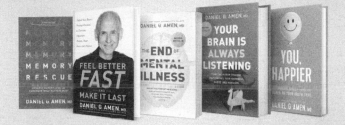